WHAT'S WRONG WITH YOU?

AN INSIDER'S GUIDE TO YOUR INSIDES

DR SARAH HOLPER

D1303295

Hardie Grant

BOOKS

Published in 2021 by Hardie Grant Books,
an imprint of Hardie Grant Publishing

Hardie Grant Books (Melbourne)
Building 1, 658 Church Street
Richmond, Victoria 3121

Hardie Grant Books (London)
5th & 6th Floors
52–54 Southwark Street
London SE1 1UN

hardiegrantbooks.com

 A catalogue record for this
book is available from the
NATIONAL
LIBRARY National Library of Australia
OF AUSTRALIA

What's Wrong with You?
ISBN 9781743797112

10 9 8 7 6 5 4 3 2 1

Edited by Geoff Slattery
Cover design by Mietta Yans
Typeset in Sabon by Kirby Jones

Printed in the US by McNaughton & Gunn,

To my parents.
Thank you for your unwavering support,
and genetic material.

CONTENTS

INTRODUCTION

I've learnt odd things working as a doctor. Interest in discussing bowel motions increases proportionally with age. Heavily tattooed people tend to be needle phobic. The phrase 'testicular trauma' will reliably cause a man to cross his legs. Then there are the procedural skills: I've learnt how to suture eyebrows back together, drill holes in skulls, and remove appendices and skin cancers. I once even learnt how to extract a receipt spike from a barista's forearm. Above all, I've learnt that everyone is fascinated by their body. What comes out of it, what can go wrong with it and why people have the symptoms they do.

Everybody has a body, and everybody gets sick. But unless you go to medical school, you're never taught how to interpret common symptoms. Why do teenagers and bodybuilders get acne? Why do you feel like yawning when you're tired, nervous, or when you think about yawning (like now)? Why do most men go bald, but women (and castrated men) don't?

Patients are often self-conscious about their lack of medical knowledge. I'm always quick to provide reassurance: why should you be expected to understand how your body works just because you have one? I have a microwave; from my perspective, it works via push-button magic. Similarly, I'm not embarrassed that I can't speak Portuguese because I've never been taught it. Some patients pretend to understand medical lingo to not look 'stupid'. Others fester with anxiety and defer medical attention because they misinterpret their symptoms as harbingers of some terminal disease (invariably cancer or a rare tropical infection).

Doctors have an unfair monopoly on body-based knowledge. Historically, we learnt anatomy by dissecting the grave-robbed corpses of criminals. Nowadays, we attend medical schools where it takes us years to learn the science of how the body functions. When we graduate, many of us forget that the intricacies of human anatomy and physiology aren't common knowledge.

Doctors think in terms of diagnoses: catch-all Latin labels that neatly account for the patient's symptoms. But patients (i.e. normal people) don't care about these impenetrable terms we commonly use like myocardial infarction, transient ischaemic attack or facioscapulohumeral muscular dystrophy (well, we don't *commonly* use that one). Most patients just want doctors to explain what's going on inside them that's causing them to feel sick. Being armed with knowledge is not only fascinating, but it helps psychologically in the recovery process.

Thankfully, medicine is rapidly shifting from the paternalistic model of 'the doctor knows best'. Hurried assurances that your symptoms are 'normal' or 'nothing to worry about' are unacceptable: you have the right to understand what's going wrong with you when you feel unwell. It's your body, for goodness' sake.

Health misconceptions plague people from all social classes, postcodes and levels of education. Shonky advice from celebrities, personal trainers and social media is taken as gospel. You wouldn't heed an actor's advice to fix your loose tap; nor should you heed their advice to fix your loose bowels. One in every 15 Google searches is health-related: that's over a billion Dr Google consultations per day. It would be better if you got the facts from a more trustworthy source (ideally one whose responses aren't influenced by an algorithm tracking your eBay purchases).

What's Wrong with You? contains plenty of those facts, plus the juicy bits from medical school and my life as a doctor, minus unpaid overtime and the smell of embalming fluid. It's packed with hospital anecdotes, cultural diversions and historical oddities. If you've ever wondered why you're dizzy, burpy, baldy, chesty, deafy or sniffy (all of which, incidentally, were brainstormed dwarf names that Walt Disney rejected for his 1937 classic *Snow White and the Seven Dwarfs*) then *What's Wrong With You?* is for you.

– Dr Sarah Holper

BRAIN

HEADACHE

The brain is the only organ that named itself. Mull over that for too long and a headache may result.

Of the skills required by a banjo player, excellent fine-motor control is perhaps the most important. An ability to tolerate widespread contempt for your craft is another. In the early 2000s, legendary American banjoist Eddie Adcock began to struggle with a tremor in his plucking hand, an ailment known as 'essential tremor'. No medication could control the potentially career-ending shaking in his right hand. 'It was probably the most devastating thing I've ever faced in my life,' Adcock admitted.

In 2008, at the age of 70, Adcock opted to undergo deep brain stimulation in an attempt to terminate the tremor. The surgeon, Dr Joseph Neimat at Tennessee's Vanderbilt University Medical Centre, drilled a hole in Adcock's skull, then skewered the exposed brain with a metal electrode. He pushed it through Adcock's brain until its tip was sitting in the thalamus, the faulty tremor-triggering region. The surgical team hoped to scramble the thalamus's tremor signal by passing an electric current through the tip of the electrode.

Banjo in hand, Adcock remained conscious during the three-and-a-half-hour procedure, treating the surgical team to (or, depending on your view of bluegrass music, subjecting them to) a private banjo concert. Adcock provided feedback on his strumming control as the surgeon adjusted the electrode's depth and level of stimulation. After meticulous millimetre and millivolt adjustments, Adcock's tremulous plucking became perfect. 'I knew when [the surgeon] had the sweet spot, and that was it,' he reported.

While the delicate procedure was painstaking for the surgeon, it certainly wasn't painful for Adcock. If you cracked open your skull and jabbed your brain with a sharp stick, you'd feel nothing. Admittedly, slicing through your scalp and removing the bone would hurt a fair bit, but the actual brain prodding would be fine. Your brain can't feel pain. It receives all the information from pain sensors around your body but has none of its own. Since slicing or impaling the brain is painless, procedures like the one that Adcock underwent can be performed with the patient awake.

Keeping the patient conscious isn't just to save money on general anaesthetic drugs. If the neurosurgeon strays into a critical region of the brain, a conscious patient can immediately make this clear (by saying 'I can't move my left foot', or 'my shpeech ishh shlurry', for example). Live feedback allows the surgeon to avoid melon-balling out functional areas of the patient's brain. If the patient were asleep, the neurosurgeon would only discover that they'd accidentally damaged a critical brain structure when the patient awoke, paralysed or mute, in the recovery room.

Some neurosurgeons prefer the 'asleep-awake-asleep' strategy: the patient is initially rendered oblivious to the rather off-putting racket and vibration of skull drilling, is conscious during the brain-fiddling, then anaesthetised again while their scalp is stitched back together. The final 'asleep' phase reduces patient anxiety, with the added benefit of allowing the surgeon to chitchat uninhibitedly about their weekend plans. I jest – neurosurgeons rarely have weekends off. Nor do they participate in chitchat.

*

Hold up two fists, as though you're about to throw a punch. Now, put your fists together with the fingernails touching. That's the rough size and shape of your brain – a 1.4-kilogram (three pound) wrinkly, beige organ responsible for everything you've ever thought, said or done. Being 75 per cent water, your brain is surprisingly squishy: the consistency of soft tofu. A fresh brain placed on a bench is liable to deform and tear due solely to the effects of gravity. Thankfully, *in vivo*, your blobby brain is supported inside your skull by your triple-ply meninges. These three layers of membranous 'cling-film' contain a cushioning fluid layer that suspends your brain to maintain its shape.

Each of the three meningeal layers has distinct characteristics. The delicate innermost meningeal layer, tenderly enveloping your brain's every wrinkle, is called your *pia mater* (Latin for 'loving mother'). The second layer sticks to the *pia mater* via cobweb-like mesh, hence it's called the *arachnoid mater* ('spider mother'). A thin layer of fluid flows in the webby space between the *pia mater* and the *arachnoid mater*. The fluid, which looks indistinguishable from water, is called cerebrospinal fluid. Anchoring the *arachnoid mater* to the skull is the third and final layer, the fibrous *dura mater* ('tough mother').

The three layers of meninges can be thought of as akin to an orange: the fine membrane over each segment, the cobwebby pith, and the tough outer peel. The slightly creepy 'mother' references come from a translation of a medical text written by the 10th century Persian physician Haly Abbas. At the time, Arabic doctors referred to the meninges as 'mothers' because they believed that these protective wrappings were the source of (i.e. the mother of) all the membranes in the body.

Since, as Eddie Adcock would attest, your brain is incapable of feeling, clearly the pain of a headache doesn't come from your brain. Alas, although the brain itself lacks pain receptors, the structures around it do not. Your *dura mater*, the muscles in your scalp, neck and face, your sinuses, eyes, teeth, ear canals, blood vessels throughout your head and the inner bony surface of your skull are all pain-sensitive. Even if you are a tough mother, anything irritating, stretching, pulling on, pushing on, infecting or otherwise damaging these structures can give you a headache.

From a doctor's perspective, there are three sorts of headaches: deadly headaches, common bread-and-butter headaches, and rare and unusual headaches. Let's consider them each in turn.

The deadly headaches

First, let's address the elephant in the room: could your headache be a brain tumour? If you've just got a headache and no other symptoms, then it's unlikely. Usually a brain tumour causes headache and other neurological problems like seizures, problems with thinking, gradual changes in behaviour or focal weakness. An isolated headache, with no other symptoms, is the presenting complaint in just two to 16 per cent of adults with brain tumours.[1]

Brain tumours cause a headache due to pressure. Your skull is a rock-like shell with a fixed volume somewhere between 1400 and 1700 millilitres (3 and 3.5 pints). Since your skull can't expand, if your brain increases in volume from anything (for example, a brain tumour, blood from a ruptured aneurysm, or a pus-filled abscess) the pressure inside your skull will increase. Headache results from various pain-sensitive structures being squashed (such as the swollen part of your brain pressing on your *dura mater*). The pain is classically worse in the morning and is often so severe that it wakes the patient from sleep. The unsettling experience of random projectile vomiting, without nausea, can occur if the brainstem's 'vomiting centre' becomes compressed (see *Nausea and vomiting*, page 185).

Extreme increases in pressure within the skull can be catastrophic. When there's no space left to expand, the brain will be left with no alternative but to extrude, like toothpaste, through the hole in the base of your skull where your spine usually emerges. Instantly lethal, this event is often referred to by the inappropriately cutesy term 'coning'.

Mountaineers will be familiar with warning signs on the ascent trail urging climbers with a headache to turn back. For over 2000 years headache has tormented those with a craving for climbing. Headache was so familiar to Silk Road travellers during the Han Dynasty (206 BC–220 AD) that high-altitude stretches of the Central Asian track were dubbed 'Great Headache Mountain' and 'Little Headache Mountain'.

Half of those who ascend over 3000 metres (10,000 feet) will get a headache. Usually it's a dull, pressing pain at the front of the head, exacerbated by movement. As you ascend, every breath contains less oxygen. Blood flow to your brain must increase up to 25 per cent to maintain normal oxygenation. Pressure builds within your skull from the extra blood volume, resulting in significant pain. Worse, the blood vessels become leaky, allowing fluid to leach into the brain itself. Your brain becomes bloated with fluid, a condition known as cerebral oedema. With all these volume increases inside your skull, it's only a matter of time before you 'cone' (unless you drown first from the same leaking phenomenon in the lungs, called pulmonary oedema).

An aneurysm is an abnormal bulging or ballooning at a weak spot in an artery. Like party balloons, aneurysms have very thin walls, making them precariously liable to pop. If a brain aneurysm bursts, the sudden excruciating pain is dubbed a thunderclap headache. Intriguingly, the sensation is almost universally described as being 'whacked over the back of the head with a baseball bat' (or a cricket bat, in Australian hospitals).

Rupture of a large aneurysm can cause catastrophic bleeding in the brain and death. During some stressful point in your life, a snooty bystander may have warned you that 'unless you calm down, you'll give yourself an aneurysm!' Besides such a comment being intensely irritating, it's also medically inaccurate. It's not entirely clear why some people form aneurysms in the first place, but you certainly can't voluntarily 'give yourself' an aneurysm by being stressed. A more precise warning would be: 'unless you calm down, your persistent high blood pressure could increase the risk of aneurysm formation according to some studies!'

The common 'bread-and-butter' headaches

Headaches are an almost universal human experience. Surveys show that 96 per cent of people experience a headache at some point in their life.[2] Almost three billion people had a tension-type headache or migraine in 2016, based on data from the Global Burden of Diseases Study.[3] The same research found 'tension-type headache' to be the third-most prevalent medical disorder in the world (after tooth decay and dormant tuberculosis infection). Migraine came in sixth place.

You know the feeling: that dull pressure squeezing both sides of your head like a vice. That's a tension-type headache. Eighty percent of people experience them. We used to call them 'tension', 'stress', 'muscle-contraction' or 'psychogenic' headaches because we thought the pain came from sustained neck muscle contractions induced by psychological stress. Further research disproving this theory caused debate among neurologists until everyone agreed to add the modifier '-type'.

The precise mechanisms behind tension-type headaches aren't clear. There might be overactive pain receptors around the head and neck, or heightened sensitivity to pain messages travelling through the spinal cord and brain. Whatever the cause, suggesting that a person with a tension-type headache 'just needs to relax' is unhelpful (and is likely to increase the tension).

A migraine is not just a bad headache: it's a particular type of headache associated with symptoms of temporary brain malfunction. Pain is merely stage three of the four-stage migraine process, which can span days. Not everyone who suffers migraine goes through all four phases; in fact, some people don't even experience the headache stage.

Up to three-quarters of 'migraineurs' experience warning symptoms a few days before the headache. Classic complaints include tiredness, poor concentration, irritability and an inexplicable need to yawn and urinate. Weird food cravings are also common: one of my patients devoured anything with chicken flavouring (she found this troubling as she was vegan); another patient's sugar cravings drove her to guzzle cordial neat from the bottle. All these symptoms arise from the hypothalamus, a deep brain structure responsible for regulating many basic bodily functions including thirst, appetite, emotional responses, body temperature (see *Fever*, page 33) and circadian rhythms (see *Jet lag and your body clock*, page 21).

In the hour before the headache kicks in, one third of migraineurs experience bizarre transient symptoms called an aura. Visual auras are the most common. Often it starts with a bright spot just off-centre of your vision that slowly expands into a shimmering crescent. Geometric shapes and zigzags dance around the expanding edge. The zigzags are called 'fortification spectra' because they resemble an aerial view of the complex moats and ramparts defending a medieval town. Slowly the crescent drifts into your peripheral vision, leaving a blind spot in its wake. Other non-visual auras include tingling that creeps along a limb, trouble finding words or weakness down one half of the body.

Auras are thought to be driven by a self-propagating wave of nerve firing rolling across the brain's surface. At the crest of the wave, nerves fire madly (making you hallucinate zigzagging lines). In its wake, exhausted nerves can't fire at all and may leave a residual blind spot. Using real-time imaging techniques on people experiencing an aura, researchers have clocked the wave rippling across the brain's surface at about three millimetres per minute.

Next comes the headache: throbbing, severe, and one-sided (the word 'migraine' comes from the Greek for 'pain in one half of the head'). Lights, sounds and movement are agonising. The sufferer often retreats to a dark room to sleep off the pain, which can last from four hours to three days, if not treated. Many factors contribute to the pain of a migraine, including that nerve-firing wave passing over the brain's surface during the aura. In their firing frenzy, nerves spurt out a concoction of pain-causing chemicals which activate pain receptors in the meninges sitting just above them. The resultant inflammation and changes in blood flow perpetuate the pain.

During the final recovery phase, the person is usually left drained and exhausted, though some people experience euphoria (in excess of the simple joy that the pain has gone).

We don't know why some people get migraines, but there's definitely a genetic component. Approximately 70 per cent of migraineurs have a first-degree relative who also gets migraines, and your risk of migraine is quadrupled if you have a relative who suffers migraine with aura.[4]

For those who do experience migraines, certain activities can set them off. Most people would enjoy a lazy weekend away in a mountain cabin, indulging in red wine and a charcuterie board by an open fire while a thunderstorm rages outside. But to a migraineur, such a sojourn sounds nightmarish. All of those activities – sleeping in, high altitude, alcohol, nitrates in meats and cheeses, smoke, storms, even weekends per se – are known migraine triggers. Other common migraine precipitants include menstruation, fasting, strong odours and stress. I treated a patient who was rendered bedbound by a migraine for two days every time she ran into her ex-boyfriend. She eventually moved interstate, where she became ex-boyfriend and headache-free.

Migraines afflict about 12 per cent of the population. Curiously, when you narrow the population down to just neurologists, more than half are migraineurs.[5] It could be that the 12 per cent figure is falsely low: many people endure their migraine symptoms and never receive an accurate diagnosis. Conversely, presumably neurologists – being brain specialists – more accurately self-identify their symptoms as a migraine, thus leading to those higher rates of diagnosis. Or perhaps junior doctors who suffer migraines are drawn to the specialty of neurology to understand their aching heads. Doctors joke that we tend to disproportionately suffer from diseases within our specialty. Cardiologists get heart attacks, oncologists get cancer, radiologists get CT scanners falling on them – so neurologists ought to get migraines. Or maybe neurologists' brains are just hurting from the constant metaphysical state of thinking about thinking.

The rare and unusual headaches

At medical school we're taught that 'when you hear hoofbeats, think of horses, not zebras'. Another similar aphorism is 'common disorders occur commonly'. Indeed, most headaches are 'horses': tension-type headaches and migraines. But occasionally those galloping hooves belong to rare and unusual headache 'zebras'. I've herded them together here.

Ice-pick headaches are characterised by intense, fleeting, stabbing pains felt around the head. Often these patients also experience other sorts of headaches like migraines. The ice pick tends to stab them where their other headaches are felt, suggesting that the pain might be due to twitchy, hypersensitive nerves randomly firing.

A numismatist is a person who collects coins; a patient with a nummular headache has a coin-sized patch of scalp that constantly hurts. Usually there's just one sore spot, but a few patients with two aching 'coins' have been reported.

Hypnic headaches, also called 'alarm clock' headaches, develop only during sleep and cause the patient to wake up. It's one of the few types of headache that occurs almost exclusively in older people, with a mean age of onset of around 60. Exercise headaches cause the whole head to throb, brought on by physical exertion particularly in hot weather or at high altitude.

Coital cephalgia is the charmingly euphemistic term for a headache triggered by sexual activity (either intercourse or masturbation). Neurologists divide the headaches into 'pre-orgasmic' – a dull ache that grows more intense with increasing sexual arousal – and 'orgasmic' – a thunderclap headache at the moment of orgasm. It's important to ensure that patients with the orgasmic subtype haven't actually burst an aneurysm in their brain. As you'll recall, aneurysm rupture also causes a thunderclap headache. Particularly worrying is the fact that up to 12 per cent of patients presenting with a ruptured aneurysm report to their doctor (quite sheepishly, in my experience) that the thunder 'clapped' during sex. Patients with repeated attacks of coital cephalgia are advised to take an anti-inflammatory tablet 30 to 60 minutes before sex. While this rather removes the spontaneity of the event, it's preferable to being rushed to hospital after every orgasm to ensure that a blood vessel in your head hasn't exploded.

The final rare and unusual headache, the cluster headache, is considered one of the most extraordinarily painful conditions a human can experience. The vicious pain has driven patients to suicide, hence their other name: 'suicide headaches'. Thankfully cluster headaches are rare, affecting about one in every 1000 people, with men five times more likely to suffer from them than women. Cluster headaches get their name because they strike in bouts: searing attacks up to eight times per day, typically for several weeks or months, separated by periods of remission lasting months or years. A particularly unfortunate 15 per cent of sufferers experience unremitting bouts that can last years.

Cluster headaches have an uncanny seasonal rhythmicity. Solstices and equinoxes are peak times. In recognition of the link, 'Cluster Headache Awareness Day' is observed every year on 21 March, the date of the Northern Hemisphere's spring equinox (23 September in the Southern Hemisphere). Cluster headaches don't just follow the calendar, they appear to have a watch. Attacks often occur at precisely the same time – to the minute – every day during a cluster. Nocturnal onset is common, turning many patients into insomniacs. The seasonal pattern and clock-like regularity of cluster headaches strongly implicate a malfunctioning body clock: the hypothalamus, responsible for your circadian rhythm. We don't know why the hypothalamus goes so badly off-script and triggers the searing pain, nor do we know why inhaled pure oxygen sometimes aborts the attack (hence the need for 'Cluster Headache Awareness Days' to promote further research).

'Being stabbed in the eye with a red-hot poker' is the curiously consistent description of a cluster headache. The pain is always just on one side of the head, around one eye. The eye starts watering and becomes bloodshot, the pupil shrinks, and the eyelid swells and droops. Snot starts streaming, but just from the nostril on the affected side of the head. Beads of sweat also form on that half of the face, which can also become flushed. These extra non-pain symptoms are due to misfiring of the autonomic nervous system, responsible for your unconscious bodily functions like how wide your pupils and blood vessels are. Restlessness and physical self-harm to the head are common. The attack lasts between 15 to 180 minutes before the pain and all the other symptoms abruptly disappear. Until the next night.

Patients suffer these repeated attacks for weeks or months at a time, robbed of sleep and living in fear of the next round of torture. Perhaps now you can understand that awful nickname, suicide headaches. Headaches, cluster headaches in particular, are more than just a pain in the head: they can cause significant, invisible suffering. The suffering is palpable in this excerpt from one man's experience with cluster headaches, published as 'The father in extremis' in the *Oxford Handbook of Clinical Medicine*:

> … I am careful not to wake the children as I make my way down the stairs. If they were to witness my nightly cluster ritual, they would never see me the same way again. Their father, fearless protector, diligent provider, crawling about in tears, beating his head on the hard wood floor. The pain is so intense I want to scream, but I never do. I go down three flights of stairs where I can't be heard and drop to my knees. I place my hands on the back of my head and lock my fingers together. I bind my head between my arms and squeeze as hard as I can in an attempt to crush my skull. I begin to roll around, banging my head on the floor, pressing my left eye with the full force of my palm. I search for the phone that has

always been my weapon of choice for creating a diversion, and I beat my left temple with the hand piece. I create a rhythm as I strike my skull, cursing the demon with each blow.[6]

SUMMARY: Your brain can't feel pain. Headache pain originates in pain-sensitive structures around the brain like blood vessels and the brain's protective lining.

AND ALSO ...

An explosive headache caused by explosives

Working closely with explosives carries significant health risks: loss of limb, loss of life, and a pounding headache. Headaches have been observed among people handling explosives since the Boer War. Some munition workers called the throbbing pain 'bang head' while others went for 'powder head'. Incidence peaked around the two World Wars when production of explosives, pardon the pun, skyrocketed. The headache-causing compounds are the organic nitrates used to make gunpowder and explosives like nitroglycerin and TNT (trinitrotoluene). These nitrates can be absorbed through the skin and enter the bloodstream. The first published description of headaches among men handling nitrates appeared in a 1910 article titled 'Nitroglycerin head':

> A man who is working in 'powder' may cause another person a great deal of misery by simply shaking hands or by permitting articles which he has been using to be handled by the other. A worker frequently carries some of the drug to his home in his clothing and may make his whole family sick. Sleeping in the same bed or the wearing of contaminated clothing will likewise produce effects.[7]

Once in the bloodstream, nitrates convert to nitric oxide which causes blood vessels all over the body to widen, including in the brain. Pressure rises within the skull due to the extra blood in the swollen blood vessels. Squashed pain-sensitive structures within the skull cause a severe, throbbing headache. Any posture that causes blood to pool in the head due to gravity, like bending forward or lying down, causes a surge of pain.

Mandatory use of protective clothing eventually led to a decline in bang head cases. These days, nitrates are prescribed as a medication. Lack of blood flow to the heart muscle can cause chest pain called angina. Taking nitrates, usually as a spray under the tongue, widens the blood vessels supplying the heart. With the extra blood comes extra oxygen, relieving the chest pain. As expected, headache is a common side effect.

Hydration and headaches

Since your brain is 75 per cent water, it's exquisitely sensitive to dehydration. Inadequate fluid intake (or excessive fluid loss, like when you're hungover) can temporarily cause your brain to slightly shrivel. As your brain contracts from your skull it tugs on the meninges, yanking on the pain-sensitive *dura mater* anchored to the bone. You experience this internal tug of war as a headache. But don't rehydrate on a mouthful of iced water too quickly or else you're in for another sort of headache: sphenopalatine ganglioneuralgia (a 'brain freeze' headache). When cold liquid gushes into your mouth it rapidly cools the blood in the vessels in the roof of your mouth. The sudden drop in temperature causes the vessels to squeeze tight, then rapidly reopen. The rebound dilation triggers pain receptors in your head. Pressing your warm tongue to the roof of your mouth usually provides enough heat to swiftly relieve the pain.

ENDNOTES

1 Hamilton, W. & Kernick, D. Clinical features of primary brain tumours: a case control study using electronic primary care records. *British Journal of General Practice*, 57 (542), 695–699 (2007).

2 Rizzoli, P. & Mullally, W. J. Headache. *The American Journal of Medicine*, 131 (1), 17–24 (2018).

3 Stovner, L. J., et al. Global, Regional, and National Burden of Migraine and Tension-Type Headache, 1990–2016: A Systematic Analysis for the Global Burden of Disease Study 2016. *The Lancet Neurology*, 17 (11), 954–976 (2018).

4 Kors, E. E., et al. Genetics of Primary Headaches. *Current Opinion in Neurology*, 12 (3), 249–254 (1999).

5 Evans, R. W., et al. The prevalence of migraine in neurologists. *Neurology*, 61 (9), 1271–1272 (2003).

6 Longmore, M. et al (Eds). *Oxford Handbook of Clinical Medicine*, 8th edition. Oxford University Press, p. 491 (2010).

7 Laws, C. E. Nitroglycerin Head. *Journal of the American Medical Association*, 54 (10), 793 (1910).

JET LAG AND YOUR BODY CLOCK

Your feet may not have a sense of rhythm, but your brain certainly does.

Jet lag is the bane of the modern traveller. But at least those seeking exotic lands no longer face scurvy, starvation, or a 90 per cent mortality rate en route to their destination. These were the grim realities confronting the 270 sailors aboard the first fleet to circumnavigate the globe, captained by Portuguese explorer Ferdinand Magellan. As the five-ship fleet departed Spain in 1519, the crew had no idea that they were embarking on a three-year voyage from hell. Mutiny broke out within months. Food shortages forced them to eat biscuit crumbs writhing with worms and soaked in rat urine.

Philippine warriors armed with bamboo spears and cutlasses gruesomely executed Magellan halfway through the expedition. Men died from murder, malnutrition and being marooned. After more than 1000 days at sea just 18 dishevelled men aboard one ship, the *Victoria*, remained. Nearly home and in desperate need of supplies, they docked at Cape Verde, a Portuguese colony some 3000 kilometres (1900 miles) south of their homeland. Antonio Pigafetta, an Italian scholar on board the *Victoria*, recounted in his diary:

> In order to see whether we had kept an exact account of the
> days, we charged those who went ashore to ask what day
> of the week it was, and they were told by the Portuguese

inhabitants of the island that it was Thursday, which was a
great cause of wondering to us, since with us it was only
Wednesday. We could not persuade ourselves that we were
mistaken; and I was more surprised than the others, since
having always been in good health, I had every day, without
intermission, written down the day that was current. But we
were afterwards advised that there was no error on our part,
since as we had always sailed towards the west, following
the course of the sun, and had returned to the same place,
we must have gained twenty-four hours, as is clear to anyone
who reflects upon it.[1]

Let's reflect upon it now. If you stand still on the Earth, you'll
see a sunrise every 24 hours. But if you're moving like Magellan's
fleet, travelling westward following the sun, each sunrise will
occur slightly more than 24 hours after the previous sunrise. Every
day – as measured by the time between two sunrises – will be a
bit longer than 24 hours. Over three years of sailing, those slight
extensions added up to one whole missed sunrise – thus one whole
missed day.

Pigafetta's discrepancy of a day posed a problem. How
could civilisation keep accurate historical records, fulfil trade
agreements or reliably celebrate birthdays if the day and date
could be changed by doing a lap of the globe? Sunrise counting
was no longer a foolproof method of tracking days in this new era
of global travel. We needed to arbitrarily decide on a demarcation
where one calendar day became the next on our ever-spinning
Earth.

In 1884, astronomers and delegates from 25 countries met
in Washington D.C. to invent the International Date Line: an
imaginary line extending between the North and the South Pole
through the Pacific Ocean. The west side of the line is always
24 hours ahead of the east: it's Monday 9 am on the left of the
line, but Sunday 9 am the moment you step to the right of the line,

for example. Travellers crossing the line must set their calendar forwards or back a day to ensure that their diary matches the 'real' global day and date. Thanks to the International Date Line, Pigafetta's diary dilemma is a thing of the past.

One discomfort Magellan's crew avoided was that of jet lag. Jet lag is a consequence of *rapid* travel: moving across the Earth too quickly for your body's biological rhythms (like your sleep-wake cycle) to adjust to the changed light-dark cycle around you. Apart from the death rate, there was nothing rapid about the crew's 1086-day voyage. As they inched west, the shifting sunrise time was so gradual that the men were oblivious to their 'lost' day until it was pointed out. Fortunately, travel speeds have improved since the 16th century.

Magellan would be gobsmacked if you told him that in 2017, Frenchman François Gabart sailed around the world in just short of 43 days. Solo. You could astound Magellan further by first explaining what a plane was, then, after ensuring he was sitting down, revealing that in 2005 one of these flying machines completed the first nonstop, unrefuelled lap of the world in just 67 hours, piloted solo by aviator Steve Fossett. Boggled by these bombshells, Magellan might experience mood swings, lose his appetite and struggle to fall asleep. Ironically, he'd be suffering the symptoms of jet lag: a modern malady caused by high-speed air travel.

Until the 20th century, humans had never travelled fast enough to necessitate a sudden body clock reset. Jet-propelled aircraft now allow us to crisscross the globe at a speed inconceivable to our ancestors. Our body clock is as unaccustomed to swiftly crossing time zones as Magellan would be to conceiving of a jet plane. Air travel opened a new chapter in human history. It also opened a new chapter in medical textbooks: a lengthy one on jet lag.

The term 'jet lag' seems to have first appeared in an article appearing in the *Los Angeles Times* on 13 February 1966. Journalist Horace Sutton suggested that:

If you're going to be a member of the Jet Set and fly off to Katmandu for coffee with King Mahendra, you can count on contracting Jet Lag, a debility not unakin to a hangover. Jet Lag derives from the simple fact that jets travel so fast they leave your body rhythms behind.[2]

By 'body rhythms' he means circadian rhythms. Sutton's unfamiliarity with the term circadian is understandable: the Romanian-American scientist Franz Halberg had only coined it in 1959. Halberg based the word 'circadian' on the Latin words *circa* and *diem*, meaning 'about a day'. His vagueness was deliberate: circadian rhythms are patterns of biological activity that repeat about every 24 hours (every 24.2 hours, on average, as we will soon learn).

Your sleep-wake cycle is the most obvious example of a circadian rhythm. Every day, two hormones called melatonin and cortisol peak and trough to make you sleepy and alert at the appropriate times. Melatonin's soporific effects prepare your body for sleep. Melatonin is made and released by your pine cone-shaped pineal gland (*pinea* is Latin for 'pine cone'), a pine nut-sized structure perched atop your brainstem. Drowsiness sets in as your blood's melatonin concentration climbs through the evening, peaking at 3 am. At this point, cortisol levels begin to rise to prepare you for waking. Cortisol readies your body for exertion by boosting your blood pressure, heart rate and blood sugar level. It's released by your two adrenal glands: fatty yellow structures resembling melted cheese draped over each kidney. By 9 am your blood cortisol levels have reached their daily maximum. Most heart attacks happen between 6 am and noon, partially due to the strain on the cardiovascular system from this morning cortisol surge.

Body temperature, digestion and the release of certain hormones also follow circadian rhythms. For example, you're hottest at 6 pm and coolest at 4 am. Intestinal squeezing and digestive juice squirting pause overnight. Instead, it's your brain's pituitary gland that's squirting out growth hormone (important for controlling your body's muscle and fat composition) and thyroid-releasing hormone (which regulates metabolism) while you sleep.

Much of our understanding of circadian rhythms comes from experiments conducted on humans in isolation. Without any external cues like clocks or daylight, what natural rhythms to their biological processes – if any – would emerge? In the 1960s, the German physician Jürgen Aschoff built an underground bunker to perform isolation experiments on volunteers. Recruitment was surprisingly straightforward, presumably because 'evil scientist with torture dungeon' was yet to become established as a horror movie trope. One at a time, subjects would enter the bunker and live alone, without watches or natural sunlight, for three to four weeks. Aschoff asked his subjects to lead a regular life. They prepared food in the bunker's small kitchen when they felt peckish. They went to bed when they were tired and woke when they felt refreshed. Aschoff wryly noted that many subjects were students who used the enforced solitude to cram for an examination. At one point, Aschoff locked himself in the bunker to try it out:

> After a great curiosity about 'true' time during the first two days of bunker life, I lost all interest in this matter and felt perfectly comfortable to live 'timeless'.[3]

Bedtimes, wake times, sleep duration and the activity of each subject were documented. A rectal probe provided continuous body temperature readings. Urine volume and electrolyte concentrations were meticulously plotted. When Aschoff examined his data a clear pattern emerged. The measured biological functions were repeating in cycles lasting 'about a day' – they were circadian. Aschoff calculated the average circadian period to be 24.9 hours (later experiments by other researchers with larger sample sizes revised the average to 24.2 hours). Aschoff's bunker experiments demonstrated that a human kept in isolation without any way of knowing the time will continue to alternate regularly between wakefulness and sleep, with other biological functions fluctuating rhythmically alongside.[4]

Pause for a moment and consider how remarkable this fact is. We live on a planet that happens to rotate at a speed that means the sun is overhead every 24 hours. By means of comparison, a day on Jupiter lasts about 10 hours while a Venusian day drags on for 5832 hours or 243 Earth days. Somehow, even when you're locked in a bunker, which could be located on Jupiter for all you know, your body's functions will still insist on operating in cycles that are roughly 24 hours long. The Earth's speed of rotation is entrenched in your DNA.

It's not some quirky cosmic coincidence: it's evolution. Animals need to do the right thing at the right time to survive. Prior to artificial lighting, human behaviour was dictated by day and night. Survival depended on maximising daytime productivity. Humans' feeble night vision, and diminished hearing and sense of smell compared with other animals, render us ill-equipped for nocturnal activities. Our ancestors who snoozed all day and stumbled about at night in search of berries did not enjoy a long lifespan. Through the process of natural selection, they developed circadian rhythms that sent them to bed at night for protection and woke them at dawn to resume fruitful activities. Their body rhythms evolved to match their home planet's 24-hour cycles of light and dark, since this gave them the best chance of survival.

By developing self-sustained internal rhythms that are in sync with our environment, we can anticipate predictable changes in our environment and prepare in advance. For example, you don't have to wait for sunrise to trigger a cortisol surge: its circadian release schedule has seen its levels rising since 3 am to peak, as required, at 9 am. Circadian rhythms, orchestrated by your body clock, allow your biological processes to be pre-emptive rather than passive.

Messing with our circadian rhythms can have serious consequences. Humans have evolved to perform at our peak during the day and sleep at night. If we're forced to perform cognitively taxing tasks when our body clock thinks it's night (due to jet lag, or night shifts, for example), the results can be disastrous. Decision-making, emotional regulation, concentration, reaction times and introspection are all impaired. Accidents and errors working with machines are more likely to happen overnight than during the day. The majority of single vehicle driving accidents occur in the hours near dawn. Early morning has also historically been the peak time for human-error catastrophes, such as the nuclear accidents at Chernobyl (1.30 am) and Three Mile Island (4 am), and the Bhopal gas leak (1 am).

*

In the wake of Aschoff's bunker experiments, the hunt for the body clock – the part of the brain responsible for orchestrating our circadian rhythms – was on. One curious finding from Aschoff's research gave scientists a tantalising tip-off about where to start their search. By fiddling with the bunker's light intensity, Aschoff found that he could prolong or contract a subject's circadian period. The body clock, it seemed, used light to wind its hands forwards or backwards. On this premise, body clock-seeking scientists homed in on areas of the brain around the optic nerves: the communication cables relaying light information from the back of each eye to the brain. In 1972, researchers inflicted brain damage on some unlucky rats and discovered that when they scrambled a part of the rats' hypothalami, just above the optic nerves, their predictable daily pattern of drinking and wheel running was abolished.[5] The researchers had successfully located (and smashed) the rats' body clocks.

Indeed, the notion of a body clock isn't just a twee metaphor: it's a physical timekeeping structure in your brain that's as tangible as your wristwatch. Your body clock sits within your hypothalamus, a key brain region responsible for regulating many basic bodily functions including thirst, appetite and body temperature. The clock takes the form of two tiny clusters of nerves, each the size of a sesame seed. The seeds sit right at the front of your hypothalamus, poised over the point where your two optic nerves meet in a cross shape. All that geographical information is crammed into your body clock's name: the suprachiasmatic nucleus. *Supra* means 'above' in Latin, *chiasm* is Greek for 'cross-shaped' (as in *chi*, the Greek letter X), and *nucleus* is Latin for 'kernel'. To save time (ironically), medical types refer to the body clock as the SCN.

Since the average circadian period is a bit over 24 hours, your SCN must routinely adjust its hands to maintain alignment with the 24-hour Earth day. It tweaks its settings based on environmental cues called zeitgebers (German for 'time givers', a term coined by Aschoff in 1960). Social interactions and meals are zeitgebers: if you're chatting with mates over a burger, for example, your SCN infers it's not bedtime. But the most potent zeitgeber, by a long shot, is light. Your SCN can't discriminate between sunlight and artificial lighting. If bright light is streaming into your eyes after sunset, your SCN deduces that it's still daytime and will prolong your circadian period. It will delay melatonin release, for example, and tell your intestines to keep squeezing. Conversely, if light floods your eyes before dawn, your SCN assumes that it's morning already and will wind its hands forwards. Cortisol levels will surge as your SCN hurries along your body's biological processes to catch up with the Earth's light and dark cycle. Unnatural light exposures like watching TV just before bed or checking your phone in the middle of the night can disrupt your circadian rhythms and cause sleep problems.

Blind people can struggle to live in sync with Earth's 24-hour rotation. Their SCN has lost its most important zeitgeber:

environmental light data from their eyes. I once had a patient who was blinded after suffering severe facial burns. After the accident he relied on speaking clocks, alarms, and his wife telling him it was bedtime to keep him on schedule. It wasn't enough: he'd lie in bed for hours, unable to sleep, as his stubborn SCN stuck to its unadjusted 24.2-ish hour circadian period. Eventually, taking melatonin tablets every evening allowed him to maintain an artificial sleep-wake pattern that matched the Earth's light-dark cycle.

*

'West is best, east is a beast' is an oft-uttered aphorism of veteran jetsetters. They're right: jet lag symptoms are often milder when travelling west compared to east. Flying west, 'back in time', requires you to prolong your circadian period to match the local clocks. Since the average circadian period is longer than 24 hours anyway, you've already got a head start. Unfortunately, that head start becomes a hindrance when travelling east, when you need to perform the usual slight truncation to 24 hours, plus further shortening to align with local time. Strategically seeking and avoiding light exposure can help your SCN to reset faster. Altering your bedtime and wake time in the days leading up to a long-haul flight can ease the transition too.

Jet lag symptoms – insomnia, daytime sleepiness, poor appetite and moodiness – occur because your bodily functions aren't happening at the appropriate time. Let's put the science into practice. Imagine you're flying west from Melbourne to Paris, heading eight hours 'back in time'. You disembark at 3 pm local time, but it's 11 pm according to your SCN, which has already coordinated your evening melatonin release and initiated intestinal shut-down. You join the locals in some afternoon tea, but as the *crêpe au citron* slips into your sleep-mode stomach you immediately feel queasy. You retire to your hotel room where the sleep pressure from melatonin becomes impossible to resist. Come 1 am and you sit bolt upright, heart pounding, the result of your SCN's 'it's 9 am in Melbourne' cortisol peak. As you watch the sun eventually rise, not having slept another wink, you can barely speak English let alone French. Your irritation is piqued by a baker snorting at your mispronounced request for a *braguette* (the zipper on your pants), which you don't feel like eating anyway.

SUMMARY: Your body clock orchestrates your circadian rhythms: cycles of biological activity that repeat about every 24 hours to match the Earth's 24-hour light-dark cycle. Jet travel lets you cross time zones faster than your body clock can adjust. Until your body clock resyncs with local time, you'll suffer jet lag symptoms.

AND ALSO ...

Hamster brain surgery

If reincarnation existed, you wouldn't want to return as a research rodent. In 1987, scientists in Cincinnati Ohio poked electrified pins into the brains of some male golden hamsters to fizzle their SCNs.[6] As expected, without a functional body clock the hamsters' circadian behavioural patterns vanished. What would happen, the scientists wondered, if they transplanted working SCNs back into these hamsters? Would their circadian rhythms return? Alas, more bad news for research rodents. The scientists killed some pregnant hamsters and harvested the SCNs from their unborn babies' brains. Working rapidly, they injected the tiny still-ticking body clocks into each male hamster's freshly fizzled brain. Post-op, astonishingly, the male hamsters returned to behaviour that followed a circadian rhythm. The body clock, it turns out, is as transferable as a wristwatch.

Waking up to reality

Sailors deployed aboard submarines say farewell to family, frolicking in open fields and natural light for months. Starting in the 1960s, naval commanders subverted this isolation to their advantage. There's no reason why submariners should follow a 24-hour day, they reasoned, besides the convention dictated by sunrise and sunset. Below the waves, days could be any duration the commander wanted. A hyper-productive 18-hour day was invented: six hours for work, six hours for meals and training drills, and a final six hours for sleep. Cutting on-duty shifts from eight to six hours aimed to limit fatigue. If a sailor zoned out while manning the sub's nuclear reactors and missiles, the consequences could be catastrophic. The crew was divided in three, with a third of the crew being in any one block at any given time. In theory, the staggered schedules ensured a constant supply of wide-awake submariners to keep watch.

Alas, the scheme – which looked flawless on paper – flopped in practice. The human circadian period is 24-ish hours. A bolshie navy commander scrubbing six hours off the clock doesn't change that fact. Data from the US Naval Submarine Medical Research Laboratory revealed that sailors consistently became fatigued every third cycle, when they would be working during the hours that their SCN had scheduled for sleep. Admitting defeat in 2014 the Navy transitioned submariners back to a regular 24-hour day. A year after the change, Commander Tony Grayson reflected on the improvement:

> ... the crew [are now] able to establish and keep their
> circadian rhythm. Imagine how you feel when you fly on
> a long flight through several time zones. This 'jet lag'
> is what we were asking our sailors to deal with every
> day by shifting their sleep 6 time zones to the east with

each [period on] watch. That schedule affected the sailors because they would often end up being wide awake when it was time to sleep.[7]

Lieutenant Travis Nicks attested to the vastly improved life aboard a 24-hour submarine:

The officer of the deck [is no longer] leaning up against the scope with both eyes closed and being slapped by the junior officer of the deck to stay awake.[8]

ENDNOTES

1   Pigafetta, A. *The First Voyage Round the World, by Magellan.* Stanley, H. E. J. (ed). Hakluyt Society (1874).

2   Maksel, R. When did the term 'jet lag' come into use? *Air & Space Magazine* (17 June 2008). https://www.airspacemag.com/need-to-know/when-did-the-term-jetlag-come-into-use-71638/#wuYyAiVATMYqzOzS.99.

3   Aschoff, J. Circadian Rhythms in Man: A self-sustained oscillator with an inherent frequency underlies human 24-hour periodicity. *Science Magazine*, 148 (3676), 1427–1432 (1965).

4   Aschoff, J. et al. Desynchronization of human circadian rhythms. *The Japanese Journal of Physiology*, 17 (4), 450–457 (1967).

5   Stephan, F. K. & Zucker, I. Circadian Rhythms in Drinking Behavior and Locomotor Activity of Rats Are Eliminated by Hypothalamic Lesions. *Proceedings of the National Academy of Sciences*, 69 (6), 1583–1586 (1972).

6   Lehman, M. N., et al. Circadian Rhythmicity Restored by Neural Transplant. Immunocytochemical Characterization of the Graft and Its Integration with the Host Brain. *The Journal of Neuroscience*, 7 (6), 1626–1638 (1987).

7   Bergman, J. Submariners on New 24-Hour Watch Schedule. *Connecticut Office of Military Affairs* (25 October 2015). https://portal.ct.gov/OMA/In-the-News/2015-News/Submariners-On-New-24-Hour-Watch-Schedule.

8   Larter, D. B. This 'life-changing' shift has made submariners much happier. *Navy Times* (28 October 2016). https://www.navytimes.com/news/your-navy/2016/10/28/this-life-changing-shift-has-made-submariners-much-happier/.

FEVER

Why some diseases make you hot under the collar.

If you had syphilis in the 1920s, your doctor may have offered to give you malaria. Until penicillin became widely available in the 1940s, syphilis had no cure. Malaria, however, was curable using quinine. Before political correctness mandated a renaming, what we now call 'late-stage syphilis' was referred to as 'general paresis of the insane'. When the syphilis infection spreads to your brain and spinal cord, it paralyses you, and makes you – well – insane. Once those symptoms set in, you have about three years left to live. Pioneered by Austrian psychiatrist Julius Wagner-Jauregg, the theory behind 'malariotherapy' was that the heat from the malarial fever would weaken the bacteria responsible for syphilis, *Treponema pallidum*. In 1917, Wagner-Jauregg drew blood from malaria-infected patients at a local hospital (mainly soldiers who had been fighting in the Balkans) and injected it directly into nine of his syphilitic patients. One died, two were sent to asylums, and six showed significant improvement (but four of them eventually relapsed). The remaining two, however, completely recovered. Encouraged, Wagner-Jauregg continued infecting his patients with malaria. In 1921 he published a case series of 200 of his malariotherapy patients, of whom 50 had recovered sufficiently to return to work.

Despite malariotherapy being reminiscent of the nursery rhyme 'The Old Lady Who Swallowed A Fly', in 1927 Wagner-Jauregg became the first psychiatrist to receive the Nobel Prize in Physiology or Medicine. Malariotherapy enjoyed a brief popularity in the early 20th century but was quickly abandoned when penicillin emerged as a less ethically dubious treatment for late-stage syphilis. Another of Wagner-Jauregg's novel ideas was to sterilise people with schizophrenia, a disorder he inexplicably attributed to masturbation. The Nobel Committee wasn't so keen on that work.

*

If you're in a pub quiz, the answer to the often-posed question: 'what is the normal human body temperature?', is 37°C (98.6°F). But this answer is as vague as the ingredients list on a can of Spam (the first being 'pork with ham'). Are they asking about core body temperature? This is your true temperature: the heat of the blood deep inside you. But since swirling a thermometer in your aorta is technically challenging, doctors tend to measure more accessible cavities. So, which site is the quizmaster asking about?

Let's say your core blood temperature was exactly 37°C. A thermometer under your tongue would read 36.5°C (97.7°F) while one under your armpit would read 36.0°C (96.8°F). A no-touch infrared thermometer aimed at your forehead should match your oral temperature, unless you've recently been blasted with freezing wind (after a wintery walk to work during the COVID-19 pandemic, my forehead temperature was often just 33°C/91.4°F). Intestinal bacteria generate heat as they digest your food, breed and go about their daily activities; hence a rectal reading is hotter than your core: 37.5°C (99.5°F). Whatever site you're measuring will fluctuate by another half degree throughout the day. At 4 am you're at your coolest; at 6 pm you're at your hottest. Thus, depending when and where you're measuring, anything from 35.5°C (95.9°F) to 38°C (100.4°F) is 'normal'. To avoid things getting heated in the pub, I suggest you just write '37°C (98.6°F)' and quietly sip your lager.

A 2017 study of over 35,000 healthy Americans, using mostly oral readings, reported an average body temperature of 36.6°C

(97.9°F).[1] Older people were colder: subjects cooled down, on average, 0.021°C every decade. Conversely, researchers found 'African-American women the hottest', their average body temperature being 0.052°C higher than white men. Note how tiny these trends are: we're talking differences in the order of hundredths of a degree. Their study highlighted just how uniform human body temperature is across ages, races and sexes: 95 per cent of people had a temperature between 35.7°C (96.3°F) and 37.3°C (99.1°F): a range of just 1.6°C (2.8°F).

Why should it be that a body temperature somewhere in the vicinity of 37°C (98.6°F) is so important? It's the balancing point of an evolutionary seesaw: hot enough to keep fungal infections at bay but not so hot that you need to eat like a bodybuilder to maintain your metabolism.

Fungi are very old, evolutionary speaking. If you compressed Earth's 4.5 billion-year existence into one calendar year, fungi would appear on November 15 while humans would arrive at 24 minutes to midnight on New Year's Eve. By the time humans hit the scene, fungi had already been evolving for millions of years to thrive at about 15°C (59°F), the Earth's average surface temperature. Very few places on Earth are as hot as a human's insides. For instance, the world's hottest cities, such as Assab and Massawa in Eritrea, boast an average annual temperature of around 30°C (86°F). Most fungal species are unaccustomed to the temperatures reached in our toasty innards: they literally can't handle the heat. As a result, warm-blooded creatures like us are only bothered by a few hundred fungal species (like *Candida* species, which cause oral thrush, and *Trichophyton* species, responsible for athlete's foot) while cold-blooded animals like reptiles and amphibians are vulnerable to tens of thousands of different fungi.

If you've ever been maddened by jock itch or a vaginal yeast infection, you're probably wondering why your body couldn't run at 47°C (116.6°F) or even 57°C (134.6°F) and prevent *all* fungal infections? The trade-off is the amount of fuel this would require.

Your body heat comes from energy in what you eat, measured in calories (from the Latin *calor* meaning 'heat'). In 2010 scientists ran a mathematical model to determine the theoretical optimal human body temperature where fungal protection was maximal, but extra food requirements needed to reach that temperature were minimal.[2] The result? 36.7°C (98.1°F), pretty damn close to the 37°C (98.6°F) that we have ended up at via evolution. It seems that 37°C is the Goldilocks zone: hot enough to make most fungi uncomfortable, but not so hot that we require constant feasting to maintain the furnace.

*

The chemical reactions that keep you alive function optimally when you're at 37°C. Everything you do – digesting, walking, thinking – happens as a result of chemical reactions. Reactions to break carbohydrates into sugars, liberate energy for muscle contraction, release and mop up neurotransmitters (the chemicals that allow messages to flow between nerves). You can conveniently refer to all these life-sustaining reactions as your 'metabolism'.

Proteins are central to your metabolism. When you hear 'protein' you probably imagine a juicy steak or those chalky 'heath bars' sold at gyms, but chemically speaking, proteins are just chains of molecules called amino acids. There are 20 different amino acids and arranging them in different orders can produce proteins as diverse as insulin, collagen in skin and bone, antibodies, haemoglobin, muscle fibres (a steak is just a cow's muscle fibres after all), and a sperm's wiggly tail.

Enzymes are proteins that accelerate (catalyse) reactions by up to a million times by forcing molecules to interact. You can rapidly extract nutrients from food thanks to digestive enzymes like lipase (which breaks down fat), lactase (lactose in dairy) and amylase (starch). You are, essentially, a bag of water and proteins. The bag – keratin in skin – is also protein. Your DNA holds the code for how to arrange amino acids to make all these different proteins. That's how important proteins are: your DNA's *sole* function is to store the recipes for how to make them.

Human proteins – and thus you – work optimally over a very narrow temperature range. Too cold and proteins stiffen up; too hot and they can permanently deform. Consider an egg white (which contains albumen, a protein) that transforms from clear slime to white rubber when it's heated. Keeping things at 37°C (98.6°F) isn't just a technique to fend off fungi: it's critical to keeping your life-sustaining chemical reactions ticking over. If those reactions stop, so do you. Permanently.

The responsibility for preventing your brain from becoming a fried egg lies with your body's thermostat: the hypothalamus. Here's a guide to finding it. Imagine inserting a skewer up one nostril. Keep inserting the skewer until you hit something squishy. You've hit your pituitary gland, responsible for squirting out various hormones like those controlling lactation (prolactin, a protein) and growth (growth hormone, also a protein). Keep stabbing for about another centimetre (half an inch). Well done! You've impaled your hypothalamus! Neurosurgeons actually use this technique to operate on the pituitary gland, though they'd probably take umbrage at my use of 'skewer' to refer to their complicated operating sticks.

Your hypothalamus constantly monitors the temperature of the blood flowing through it. It also receives peripheral temperature intel from receptors in your skin. If your temperature is deviating from 37°C, your hypothalamus intervenes to bring things back to normal.

If you're getting cold, the first step is to conserve whatever heat you already have. The hypothalamus sends nerve signals to tiny muscles beneath the hairs in your skin, instructing them to contract. Upon pulling taut, the muscles yank up the overlying hair, causing it to stand on end in a process called piloerection. You see the tensed muscles beneath the skin as goosebumps. By trapping air, the erect hairs maintain an insulating warm air layer against your skin (this technique worked better for our shaggy primate ancestors, but evolutionary responses die hard). Your hypothalamus also sends nerve impulses to blood vessels near your skin's surface, squeezing them closed to reroute blood deeper within you. This minimises radiant heat loss: your toes and fingers might turn white and freeze, but at least your heart won't. Hypothalamus-initiated behavioural changes, like a desire to seek shelter and don more clothing, further promote heat conservation.

Having saved what heat you have, the second weapon in your hypothalamus's arsenal is heat generation. Rapid muscle contractions like shivering and teeth chattering make heat via kinetic (movement) energy. These actions are more effective at producing heat than exercise like running, since you remain still. If you started jogging, you'd lose heat via radiation from exposed swinging arms and legs. All these responses will continue until your hypothalamus senses that your blood has warmed back up to 37°C (98.6°F).

Now consider what happens in the opposite situation. Your hypothalamus notices that it's being bathed in blood that's too hot, say, 39°C (102.2°F). You need to cool down. Most of your hypothalamic responses here are the reverse of the 'make me warmer' ones: your skin hairs lie flat to avoid trapping heat, your superficial blood vessels dilate (hence flushed red skin), and you want to strip off and stay still, preferably in an air-conditioned room. Maximising your surface area by lying spread-eagled allows more heat to radiate into the environment.

Elephants' jumbo ears serve as giant radiators: two high surface area flaps laced with blood vessels which can wave in the breeze to offload heat. Being such chunky animals living in sweltering environments, this method of heat regulation is crucial to their survival.

Under your hypothalamus's orders, your sweat glands will start seeping out sweat. On your skin, evaporation – the process of liquid changing to a vapour – absorbs heat energy. Humans tend to use perspiration as the evaporating liquid, but other animals are more creative: overheating turkey vultures urinate on their legs, while hot bees spit in each other's faces. Perspiring is an issue for astronauts because in zero gravity, sweat just balls up on their skin and won't drip away. Wiping it off generates floating sweat beads which can lodge in the craft's sensitive equipment. To avoid short-circuits, the ambient temperature on spaceships is carefully regulated to minimise perspiration.

The 'make me warmer' script can be lifesaving if you find yourself scantily clad, caught in a blizzard with a rapidly plummeting body temperature. But sometimes heating up when you're not cold – when you're already 37°C (98.6°F) – can be lifesaving too. This is what a fever is: when your hypothalamus forces your body to run at a temperature in excess of 37°C.

In his 1666 book *The Method of Curing Fevers*, English physician Thomas Sydenham (who coined the aphorism 'first do no harm') described fever as 'nature's engine which she brings into the field to remove her enemy'. He was spot-on.

When your immune system is fighting an infection, it pumps out chemicals called pyrogens, from the Greek for 'fire-generating' (from the same root as 'pyromaniac' meaning 'fire frenzy'). Pyrogens travel through your bloodstream, eventually flowing past your hypothalamus. When your hypothalamus sees a pyrogen, it winds up the thermostat, resetting your body's target temperature at, say 39°C (102.2°F). Your current temperature of 37°C is no longer normal: it's 2°C (nearly 4°F) too cold! Shivering and goosebumps follow as the 'heat up' script plays out.

As your immune system wins the battle it stops releasing pyrogens. Your hypothalamus's set point soon drops to normal: 37°C. What happens next? Yep, you guessed it – it plays the 'cool down' script. In a flurry of perspiration and flushed skin, before long you've cooled back down to 37°C.

Fever is beneficial for two main reasons: it makes your immune system zippier, plus invading bugs become woozy and weak in the heat.

Many chemical reactions happen faster at higher temperatures. Heat provides kinetic energy: an extra oomph to let particles move faster and get to the required outcome quicker. Imagine dropping a sugar cube into a glass of iced tea. Eventually it will dissolve as water molecules bump into sugar molecules. But drop a sugar cube into hot tea and it will begin to dissolve instantly. When heated, water and sugar molecules move faster. Speedier molecules collide – and thus react – more often. The immune system is a complex series of chemical reactions. Heat it and it will work faster. Warmed white blood cells are deployed faster, travel around the body faster, devour microorganisms faster and multiply faster. So long as the temperature increase is only a few degrees (not fried-egg level: things get dicey above 42°C/107.6°F) then your body's proteins can handle the heat.

Some disease-causing pathogens become slovenly and dysfunctional at higher temperatures. For example, at fever temperatures influenza A viral replication is inhibited while some of *Salmonella** *enterica's* infective features are thwarted and it can retreat into hibernation.[3]

Part of the reason that malariotherapy sometimes worked is because *Treponema pallidum,* the syphilis-causing bacteria, are heat-sensitive. Successful infection requires a bug to breed rapidly and disperse quicker than your immune system can kill it. Even if your fever only stymies the invasion rate by a few per cent, that might be enough to inhibit infection taking hold.

Friendly bacteria living in and on you evolved to function optimally at normal human temperatures. For example, intestinal *E. coli* families and skin-based *Staphylococci* societies breed fastest

---

* *Salmonella*, despite readily infecting raw salmon, isn't named after the fish. It's actually named after Daniel Salmon (1850–1914), an American veterinary surgeon who isolated the bacteria in hogs.

at 37°C (98.6°F). Contained in the intestine and skin, they're harmless, but if they enter your bloodstream (from a ruptured intestine or deep flesh wound, for example), they can make you gravely unwell. Launch a fever however, and the subsequent sauna stymies their attack.

The fastest way to generate pyrogens is through infection, particularly with toxin-generating bacteria like *Clostridium* species (responsible for botulism, tetanus and gas gangrene), *Shigella dysenteriae* (the cause of dysentery) and *Salmonella enterica* (which causes typhoid fever). In 1969, scientists in America recruited 'volunteer' prisoners from the Maryland House of Correction to study the dose of *Salmonella* toxin required to cause a fever.[4] I wonder how 'voluntary' participation really was, since step one of the experiment was to insert a thermometer an eye-watering 15 centimetres (six inches) into the volunteer's rectum. The subjects were then 'confined to bed and covered with a light blanket' before being injected with *Salmonella* toxin of various concentrations. Within three hours, men started complaining of 'moderately severe headaches' and 'chilliness' as they developed fevers 1.4°C above baseline. What dose had they received? A minuscule 0.0014 micrograms per kilogram. Assuming an 80 kilogram (176 pound) man, that means a dose of just 0.112 micrograms caused a fever. For perspective, an eyelash weighs 40 micrograms. The prisoners' respect for the law might have been lacking, but their hypothalamic responses to pyrogens certainly weren't.

The ideal fever response is brief: it enhances your immune response then quickly withdraws once your immune system has won the battle. But what happens if your immune system doesn't win the battle? An active immune system for any reason – fighting an infection, inflammation, or cancer – will release pyrogens. An unremitting fever is an ominous sign of underlying disease. Consider some more results from that large temperature study of Americans I mentioned earlier. All the participants were seemingly healthy, without any symptoms of infection or cancer. But for every 0.149°C increase in body temperature above the expected level (accounting for variables like age and ethnicity), a person's chances of dying in the next 12 months increased by 8.4 per cent. Something bad was driving that low-grade pyrogen generation: a cancer perhaps, or a grumbling deep-seated infection. A persistent fever suggests a struggling – and failing – immune response. If your immune system loses that struggle, you die.

It is for this reason that the song 'Fever', popularised in 1958 by jazz songstress Peggy Lee, inspires fear in any doctor who hears it, especially these lines: 'You give me fever / When you kiss me / Fever when you hold me tight / Fever! In the morning / Fever all through the night'.

Night sweats are never normal. Remember, you should be at your coldest at 4 am. The loss of that natural dip suggests constant pyrogen production from a battling immune system. To distinguish true night sweats from just having too many blankets on, trainee doctors are taught to ask: 'Do you get so sweaty that you could wring out your pyjamas in the morning?' I prefer to ask patients if they could wring out their bed sheets, ever since one elderly man informed me, with a wink, that he slept in the nude.

Unintentional weight loss is another sign of a struggling immune system. Cancers and infections need energy to grow; they get that energy by breaking down your tissue stores. Energy is required to keep that fever burning, too. Tuberculosis was once called 'consumption' for the infection's notorious tendency to consume the patient's fat and muscle until their coughing skeletal body finally succumbed.

*

So, what should you do if you have a fever?

In modern times, an irate person might be told to, 'take a chill pill', but in the late 19th century this was actual medical advice given to feverish patients. 'Chill pills' principally contained quinine (which could help if you had malaria) with combinations of black pepper or powdered capsicum. The ironic inclusion of something 'hot' seemed crucial to the recipe. Paracetamol is a modern chill pill that actually does reset your hypothalamus back to 37°C (98.6°F) when you've got a fever. 'But hold on,' you say, 'given fever's benefits, surely this interference is harmful!' Logically, yes. But rigorous real-world studies have found no harm in dampening a fever.

The largest such study was performed in 2015 on 700 Intensive Care Unit (ICU) patients with fevers of at least 38°C (100.4°F).[5] Compared to the placebo group, the average temperature of those who received paracetamol was 0.28°C lower. The final result? No difference in death rates, time in ICU or total admission length.

How can we explain this? Maybe these patients were already too sick. Fever only offers a small benefit: enough to offer a survival advantage on an evolutionary timescale, but perhaps not enough to make a difference to a critically ill person dying from multi-organ failure in an ICU.

The current advice is that taking medications like paracetamol to reduce your fever is harmless. Conversely, don't attempt to cure your syphilis by injecting yourself with the blood of a malaria-infected soldier, or to castrate yourself if you have schizophrenia. Penicillin and antipsychotics, respectively, should definitely be tried first.

SUMMARY: Your hypothalamus is your body's thermostat. When you have a fever, it's because your hypothalamus has increased its set point in response to pyrogens – chemicals released in the setting of infection, inflammation or cancers. The extra heat makes your immune system stronger, and invading bugs weaker, improving your chances of recovery.

AND ALSO ...

Heatstroke vs fever

'The Human Torch' was the nickname given to Willie Jones, a 52-year-old man discovered unconscious inside his airless apartment during the 1980 Atlanta heatwave. His temperature? A mind-melting 47°C (116.6°F). Upon reaching hospital he was immediately packed in ice while icy water was pumped through him via a stomach tube in a drastic attempt at cooling his body. Remarkably, Willie recovered and still holds the not-so-hotly-contested world record for the highest-ever survived body temperature.

Hyperthermia or 'heatstroke' is not the same as fever. In fever, your body's temperature set point is deliberately increased. In heatstroke the set point is unchanged: external factors have heated you up, but your hypothalamus, despite all its tricks, has failed to cool you down. Children left in cars, endurance athletes and heavily clad members of the military are particularly vulnerable to heatstroke. The drug ecstasy can cause heatstroke because it blocks your skin's superficial blood vessels from dilating, eliminating radiant heat loss as a cooling technique. Plus, ecstasy users are often fervently dancing (which generates more heat) in crowded nightclubs with poor ventilation (which prevents sweat from evaporating).

Medical terms to heat up your vocabulary

A 'hectic fever' is one that shows wild variation between the temperature's peak and trough. Such a pattern is often seen in people with abscesses (balls of pus) festering inside them. Other fevers are 'remittent': your temperature rises and falls each day but always remains higher than normal (seen in patients with pneumonia, and many viral infections, for example). Typhoid causes a so-called 'ascending remittent fever', where your temperature rises stepwise. 'Relapsing' fevers last days, followed by days of normal temperature (characteristic of Hodgkin's lymphoma, for example). A fever that happens precisely every 21 days is seen in a rare genetic blood disorder called cyclic neutropaenia (cycles of low white blood cell levels). Fluctuating rates of white blood cell production in the bone marrow cause this unusual three-weekly pattern. Polio causes a 'saddleback' fever: a spike, then a drop before another period of fever. Trace this pattern on a graph and the saddleback name becomes self-explanatory.

Incidentally, while on saddles and polio, a horse was used in an early failed attempt to produce a polio vaccine. Researchers gave monkeys polio, dissected their spinal cords, passed the mashed cord through a sieve then repeatedly injected increasing quantities of spine mash into a horse. The horse became both cranky and immune to polio. While the horse's blood showed antiviral properties in the lab, as a human vaccine it failed miserably. Ultimately, a vaccine was developed that omitted the laborious monkey spine-mashing horse-irritating palaver.

Honey, I melted the kids

Asian giant hornets can decimate a Japanese honeybee hive in minutes. Honeybee stingers are too stumpy to pierce a hornet's thick exoskeleton. But Japanese honeybees have developed an alternative ninja skill: forming a 'hot defensive bee ball'. The kinetic energy of swarming, vibrating spheres of Japanese honeybees can buzz-up heats of 47°C (116.6°F), enough to literally cook the invading hornet alive. Less destructively, honeybees also use their body heat to mould their beeswax into hexagons.

A focus on fever frequency

Several parasite species can cause malaria. Disease severity (and your chances of survival) depends on which species was in the mosquito's saliva when it bit you. Part of the parasite's life cycle involves reproducing within your red blood cells. Once there's a full house within the cell, the parasite family bursts free, rupturing the red blood cell and triggering a massive immune response with pyrogens and fever. Different malaria-causing parasite species reproduce, burst and thus cause fever at different rates. Before we had microscopes that allowed us to visually identify the parasite species, doctors used fever patterns to diagnose and prognosticate.

Doctors could reassure patients who got a fever every third day: the mildest form of malaria is caused by a lazy species (*Plasmodium malariae*) that takes a leisurely 72 hours between bursting cycles. The prognosis for patients with fevers on alternate days wasn't too bad either: the two parasites that cause less severe malaria (*Plasmodium vivax* – the one Wagner-Jauregg infected his syphilis patients with – and *Plasmodium ovale*) have 48-hour reproductive cycles. But things looked grim for patients who got a fever one morning, then another late the next day. The parasite responsible for the deadliest form of malaria (*Plasmodium falciparum*) takes 36 hours between rupture cycles. Unfortunately, *falciparum* malaria progresses so rapidly that patients often didn't survive the several days required to observe this fever pattern.

Your chances of surviving malaria were even lower before the days of quinine, when the treatment for malaria was to say 'abracadabra'. The first recorded instance of that word was in a 3rd century text advising feverish patients to jot down 'abracadabra' multiple times on a piece of paper, omitting a letter each time until one letter remained. The paper would then be worn as an amulet around the neck for nine days before being tossed in an eastward flowing river. And you thought Wagner-Jauregg's ideas about schizophrenia and masturbation were mad?

What's good for the goose

The term 'goosebumps' derives from the skin's resemblance to that of a freshly plucked goose. But pluck any bird and the same stippled effect results. Why English favoured the goose is a mystery. Other languages are less goose-centric. The Japanese go for the all-inclusive 'bird skin'. Hebrews refer to 'duck skin'. 'Hen skin' is used in French, Spanish and Romanian, while the Dutch prefer the non-gender specific 'chicken skin'. *Horripilation* is the medical term for goosebumps. The word comes from Latin *horrere* meaning 'to bristle with fear, shudder'. The English words 'horror' and 'horrid' stem from the same origin.

ENDNOTES

1   Obermeyer, Z., et al. Individual differences in normal body temperature: longitudinal big data analysis of patient records. *British Medical Journal*, j5468 (2017).

2   Bergman, A., Casadevall, A. Mammalian Endothermy Optimally Restricts Fungi and Metabolic Costs. *mBio*, 1 (5) (2010).

3   González Plaza J. J., et al. Fever as an Important Resource for Infectious Diseases Research. *Intractable and Rare Disease Research*, 5 (2), 97-102 (2016).

4   Greisman, S. E., & Hornick, R. B. Comparative Pyrogenic Reactivity of Rabbit and Man to Bacterial Endotoxin. *Experimental Biology and Medicine*, 131 (4), 1154–1158 (1969).

5   Young, P., et al. Acetaminophen for Fever in Critically Ill Patients with Suspected Infection. *New England Journal of Medicine*, 373 (23), 2215–2224 (2015).

YAWNING

**Pandiculation describes the act of simultaneously
yawning and stretching. Just reading that fact
is likely to induce pandiculation. But why?**

Between 2007 and 2013, the US Transport Security Administration
(TSA) spent close to one billion dollars on the 'SPOT' program
(Screening of Passengers by Observation Techniques) designed to
identify potential terrorists among people milling around airports.
TSA agents were trained to recognise 92 behaviours that warranted
a pat-down and further screening. Seemingly devised by a *Loony
Tunes* enthusiast, some of the behaviours on the list (which was
leaked in 2015) included:

- Obvious 'Adam's apple' jump when requested to submit to
  screening procedures.
- Whistling as the individual approaches the screening process.
- Cold penetrating stare or widely open staring eyes.
- Excessive laughter.
- Appears to be in disguise.
- Exaggerated yawning as the individual approaches the screening
  process.

The possession of certain 'unusual items' also raised suspicion,
including the laughable Hollywood cliché: 'photographs/diagrams
of high-profile targets'. So, if you're a giggling, false beard-

wearing terrorist attempting to pass through airport security while nonchalantly whistling and gulping – beware. In 2013, the Government Accountability Office advised the TSA to 'limit future funding support' to the SPOT program after its investigations concluded that 'the human ability to accurately identify deceptive behaviour based on behavioural indicators is the same as or slightly better than chance'.[1]

Yawning seems like an odd inclusion to the TSA's list of suspicious behaviours. True, it's probably challenging to get a good sleep the night before a terrorist attack. But surely once you're in the airport, the stress would be sufficient to stifle a yawn? Or so you'd think. From the 'science' of behavioural profiling, let's turn to the similarly murky science of yawning.

Yawning is a semi-voluntary, semi-reflexive behaviour. Most people can force out a yawn on command (try it). Voluntary sneezing, however, isn't possible: sneezing is entirely reflexive. But at other times yawning *is* a reflex – an action that's out of your voluntary control. We've all stifled yawns during mundane meetings. As is often the case in neurology, patients with brain damage have provided clues about the nerve pathways that result in a yawn.

In 1923 the British neurologist Sir Francis Walshe was tending to some hemiplegic patients. Paralysed down one side of the body, their arm and leg on that side were dead weights. Until they yawned. During those glorious six or so seconds, the muscles in their paralysed limbs woke up, allowing them to stretch. Walshe concluded that an area of the brain beyond our conscious control must coordinate yawning. Although the patient couldn't voluntarily raise their arm or splay their fingers, during a yawn, alternate involuntary nerve pathways permitted the reflexive movement. 'Indeed,' reported Walshe, 'one man added that he always waited for a yawn so that he might exercise his fingers in this way.'

Yawning is not just restricted to humans – it's a widespread behaviour across the animal kingdom. Both cold-blooded and warm-blooded animals yawn. Flying, swimming and terrestrial animals yawn. Frogs yawn. Birds yawn. Fish yawn. Tortoises yawn. The naturalist Charles Darwin recognised the implications of yawning's pervasiveness: 'Seeing a dog and horse and man yawn, makes me feel how much all animals are built on one structure.' If so many animals yawn, perhaps they all evolved from a common yawning ancestor, Darwin mused. And, if so many creatures yawn, he reasoned, it must serve some important function.

Watch any species yawn and the procedure will look pretty similar. Powerful mouth opening, head tilted back, slow, deep inhalation. At peak yawn the mouth is maximally gaped, the lungs are at full capacity, the lips are drawn back, the teeth are exposed, and the eyes are scrunched shut. The heart rate and blood pressure increase. With a brief exhalation the mouth snaps shut, all the involved muscles relax, and the yawn is complete. Yawning stretches the diaphragm plus muscles in the face, neck and chest wall (plus arm muscles, if you're really committed). Be it a yak or a macaque or a horse or dog, all yawning animals follow the same script.

So why do we do it?

Scientists have been asking that question for millennia. Ancient Greek physician Hippocrates (born 460 BC) suggested that a yawning mouth functioned as a pressure valve to expel 'hot air' in patients with fever:

> Yawning precedes a fever, because the large quantity of air that has accumulated ascends all at once, lifting with the action of a lever and opening the mouth; in this manner the air can exit with ease … Like the large quantities of steam that escape from cauldrons when water boils.[2]

The French physician Jean Fernel (1497-1558) agreed with the 'gas release' idea, suggesting that yawning existed 'to evacuate harmful vapours'.

Other medics offered yawning theories that implicated four bodily fluids called 'humours' – black bile, yellow bile, phlegm and blood – whose imbalance was thought to cause disease. Reflecting on how yawning involves deep inhalation and limb stretching, the Dutch physician and botanist, Herman Boerhaave (1668–1738) proposed that yawning served:

> ... to move all the humours of the body through all the
> vessels, to accelerate their movement, to distribute them
> equally and as a result, to give the sensory organs and
> muscles of the body the capacity to perform their functions.[3]

Once doctors got over the humour-based hypotheses, another humorous suggestion emerged: we yawn because our brain needs oxygen. Dutch doctor Johannes de Gorter (1689–1762) first mooted the 'low oxygen' idea in his 1755 book *De Perspiratione Insensibili*.[4] It seems superficially logical: if your blood oxygen levels were low, a reflex that forced you to take a huge gulp of air would be useful, right?

Headed by American psychologist and neurobiologist Robert Provine, researchers in 1987 decided to test this hypothesis.[5] Remember that breathing involves inhaling oxygen and breathing out carbon dioxide. If you're not breathing quickly or deeply enough, blood oxygen levels fall and carbon dioxide levels rise. Using college students as guinea pigs, scientists measured the students' baseline yawning rate in room air (which is 21 per cent oxygen). Next, they made the students breathe 100 per cent oxygen. If the 'low oxygen causes yawning' hypothesis were true, the over-oxygenated students should stop yawning, or at least yawn less. But they didn't. Undeterred, the researchers tried the reverse: forcing the students to inhale high concentrations of carbon dioxide. This would simulate the scenario of under-breathing, where carbon dioxide accumulates in the blood. Alas, no barrage of yawning ensued. Finally, the students were asked to exercise until they doubled their breathing rate. Surely their high oxygen demands would trigger a yawn storm? Nope. It's an attractive explanation, but the idea that we yawn to suck more oxygen is a myth.

Perhaps the clue to yawning's function is revealed by those moments when humans and other animals yawn? In humans, peak yawn rates occur just before going to bed, after waking, and during tedious activities. But nervous yawning – à la those potential terrorists – is also a well-documented entity. Paratroopers often stifle a yawn prior to their first jump. Elite athletes and musicians commonly yawn before performances. Speed skater Apolo Ohno was criticised for his apparently nonchalant attitude and poor sleep routine when he was filmed yawning pre-event at the 2010 Vancouver Winter Olympics. He countered the criticism with a simple explanation: 'I kind of like it, like a lion.' Indeed, lions do like yawning, particularly. after waking from their afternoon siesta before their evening hunt. Pet dogs with a consistent daily walk schedule often start yawning even before their owner has reached for the leash. Baboons, guinea pigs and the boxer Mike Tyson have all been observed yawning when preparing to fight.

The common thread to all these yawn-inducing activities? A need to increase mental alertness in anticipation of an important event (such as an Olympic final, or a heavyweight title fight), or during a behavioural transition (from napping to gazelle hunting, or from confinement indoors to loping in a park, for example). Perhaps yawning serves to perk up our brain? This is the general consensus of modern yawn researchers.

Exactly how yawning increases mental efficiency and promotes arousal remains hazy. Maybe yawning swirls cerebrospinal fluid around the brain, helping to clear accumulated waste chemicals? Maybe yawning, by increasing your blood pressure and heart rate, causes a surge of fresh glucose-filled blood to the head, providing energy to fuel the brain's activities? Or maybe yawning keeps you on the ball by maintaining your brain's optimal operating temperature?

The 'brain-cooling hypothesis' suggests that yawning offsets transient increases in your brain's temperature. Yawning could cool down your noggin by a few different mechanisms. First, ambient air flowing through your nostrils during a yawn could physically cool the overlying brain, while the air rushing through your moist airways could offer evaporative-cooling benefits. Second, the yawn-induced rush of blood to your skull could introduce cooler blood from your peripheries. Finally, pandiculation (that exaggerated arm stretching during yawning) might promote peripheral cooling via radiant heat loss from your limbs held akimbo in the breeze. The brain-cooling hypothesis might account for why yawning escalates in the evening: at 6 pm your body, including your brain, is at its daily temperature peak. As for yawning in the morning, this could keep your brain's temperature steady while the body's metabolic processes are rapidly firing up.

In short, nobody knows why we yawn. 'Yawning may have the dubious distinction of being the least understood common human behaviour' lamented yawn expert Professor Robert Provine, the researcher who ran that seminal 1987 study debunking the yawning gets oxygen in hypothesis.[6] Yawning has many consequences – inflating your lungs, moistening your eyes, opening your eustachian tubes (see *Earache*, page 77), increasing your heart rate and blood pressure, perhaps cooling your brain – but these may be completely incidental to yawning's mysterious underlying function. Provine's best summary, after years of yawn research? Yawning 'stirs up our physiology and it plays an important role in shifting from one state to another'.[6]

It turns out that some 250 years before Provine's stirring up our physiology conclusion, two French physicians had, separately, already mooted the idea. The first was Jean-Férapie Dufieu in 1763:

When we wake, we yawn, stretch our arms, we are more agile, our spirit is more vivacious. Since the nervous juices do not flow through the muscles during sleep, all fibres are sluggish. Thus, we have to contract them all, to open the passage for the nervous juices that have filtered into the brain, or to bring them into these parts. In addition, since the movement of blood through the muscles is sluggish, its course has to be hastened; this is done by contraction where the muscles enter when the limbs are stretched. Yawning has the same cause. These nervous juices that enter into the muscles, and that have gathered up in large quantities, make us more agile, because the soul can send a large amount into the nerves to move the body parts.[7]

Five years later, François Boissier de Sauvages likewise noticed how following a yawn:

> … the soul experiences a sort of exquisite pleasure, and the person becomes more energised and more alert.[8]

We no longer talk in terms of 'nervous juices' or the soul's 'exquisite pleasure', but the gist of these Frenchmen's hypotheses is remarkably similar to the stance of modern yawn researchers.

*

There's one final quirk of yawning to add to its mystery: yawning is contagious. We yawn when we see other humans yawning. Contagious yawning has been recognised for centuries. The Dutch chemist and physician Jan Baptista van Helmont (1577–1644) pondered:

> Why do we yawn in spite of ourselves when someone else yawns? This demonstrates that yawning does not proceed from sooty vapours, but from the imagination.[3]

Humans and our closest relatives – chimpanzees – are the only animals that are susceptible to contagious yawning. Pack animals like lions and wolves have been observed yawning around the same time as each other, but there's no clear evidence that they're catching it from each other. Instead, they all seem to be individually responding to the same stimulus, such as preparing to hunt.

Contagious yawning in chimps isn't as clear-cut as it is among humans. While video experiments can induce contagious yawning in research chimps, wild chimps haven't been observed catching yawns. It's thought that the laboratory conditions used to test chimps (video loops of chimps yawning multiple times) represent a 'supernormal stimulus' that forces out contagious yawn behaviour.

In humans, seeing, hearing or even thinking about yawning can trigger a yawn. In one of Provine's studies of contagious yawning, 55 per cent of subjects yawned while watching a five-minute video of a man repeatedly yawning, compared to a yawn rate of only 21 per cent among those who watched a control video (featuring a cheerful chap repeatedly grinning).[9] If you've yawned excessively while reading this chapter, you're not alone: in another of Provine's experiments, 30 per cent of subjects asked to read an article about yawning stifled a yawn, compared to 11 per cent in the control group (who enjoyed an article about hiccoughing).

Contagious yawning is part of a phenomenon that psychologists call mental state attribution – the ability to infer, or empathise with, what others are thinking. Catching a yawn requires empathy. The more empathy you feel towards a person, the more contagious you'll find their yawns. You're more likely to 'catch' a yawn from your best friend than a random person in the supermarket, and people who score highly on questionnaires measuring empathy traits are more prone to catching a yawn. Conversely, those who struggle to understand what others are thinking and feeling, a feature of schizophrenia and autism spectrum disorders, for example, display much lower rates of contagious yawning.

A neat experiment in 2003 demonstrated the age at which kids start catching yawns.[10] Children aged from two to 11 years old watched a video of an adult mindlessly chatting about a trip to the zoo and reading nursery rhymes, while frequently pausing to yawn. Would seeing and hearing the yawns set the kids off? What about just thinking about yawns? To test this, the children then read a story (or had it read to them) that featured a yawning lead character. The results? Seen and heard, or just thought about, yawns were not contagious to any kids aged under five. Between age five and ten, rates of contagious yawning steadily climbed before plateauing at about 55 per cent (the same rate seen amongst the adults in Provine's study) among 11 years olds.

Although human embryos yawn reflexively from the 14th week of gestation, it takes us at least five years before we develop the social skills required to empathise with another person and catch their yawn. And so far, it has taken humans 2500 years – and still counting – to work out why we yawn in the first place.

SUMMARY: Yawning is a behaviour that may serve to boost mental arousal. Catching someone's yawn acknowledges their mental state and is thought to forge social bonds.

AND ALSO ...

Yawning and a different kind of 'arousal'

Decreased sex drive is a common and distressing side effect of many antidepressant medications. Yet one antidepressant has the opposite effect: clomipramine has been reported to trigger yawn-induced orgasms. A 1983 paper documented several startling patient experiences.[11] One woman 'sheepishly admitted that she hoped to take the medication on a long-term basis' because 'every time she yawned she had an orgasm. She found she was able to experience orgasm by deliberate yawning'.

Another woman complained of 'yawning spells' associated with irresistible 'sexual urges'. One man wasn't so keen to continue taking clomipramine 'because he had noted a frequent intense urge to yawn without tiredness and that on many occasions when he yawned, he experienced orgasm, with ejaculation'. He ultimately chose to keep taking the antidepressant because his mood had improved, and 'the awkwardness and embarrassment was overcome by continuously wearing a condom'.

Try to spot a giraffe yawning

Giraffes are the only mammals that haven't been observed to yawn. American psychologist and yawning researcher Ronald Baenninger had one of his graduate students watch 35 hours of zoo giraffe footage in 1992. Not a single yawn. To push blood against gravity up their 1.8-metre (5.9-foot) neck, giraffes have a resting heart rate of 170 beats per minute plus double the blood pressure we do. All those yawning hypotheses that involve increasing blood flow to the head – to provide glucose, flush out waste chemicals, cool the brain, or something else – are probably superfluous for giraffes. Since they've already got a high-pressure circulatory system running at maximum, giraffes are hardly going to benefit from the tiny extra blood flow achieved by yawning. Or maybe giraffes only yawn in private.

ENDNOTES

1   Aviation Security: TSA Should Limit Future Funding for Behavior Detection Activities. *U.S. Government Accountability Office*, 14-159 (2013).
2   Coxe, J. R. *The Writings of Hippocrates and Galen Epitomized from the Original Latin Translations. Vol: Of Flatus.* Philadelphia, Lindsay and Blakiston (1846).

3   Walusinski, O. (Ed.). *The Mystery of Yawning in Physiology and Disease.* Frontiers of Neurology and Neuroscience. S. Karger AG (2010).

4   Gorter, de J. *De Perspiratione Insensibili* (ed. 2) Italica, Manfrè Imp. Patavii (1755).

5   Provine, R. R., et al. Yawning: No effect of 3–5% CO2, 100% O2, and exercise. *Behavioral and Neural Biology*, 48 (3), 382–393 (1987).

6   Martin, R., Trudeau, M., & Provine, R. Yawning may promote social bonding even between dogs and humans [Radio broadcast]. *National Public Radio* (15 May 2017). https://www.npr.org/transcripts/527106576.

7   Dufieu, J. F. *Traité de physiologie.* Lyon, Jacquenod Fils. Lib. (1763).

8   Boissier de La Croix de Sauvages, F. *Nosologica methodica sistens morborum classes.* Amstelodami, Fratrum de Tournes (1768).

9   Provine, R. R. Yawning. *American Scientist*, 93, 532–539 (2005).

10 Anderson, J. R. & Meno, P. Psychological influences on yawning in children. *Current Psychology Letters,* 11 (2003).

11 Mclean, J. D., et al. Unusual Side Effects of Clomipramine Associated with Yawning. *The Canadian Journal of Psychiatry*, 28 (7), 569–570 (1983).

HEAD

BALDING

**'To brush one's hair' is an unusual phrase. Surely it ought
to be one's 'hairs'? Unless, alas, you are balding.**

As Julius Caesar's empire was expanding, his hairline was rapidly
receding. '[Caesar's] baldness was a disfigurement which troubled
him greatly,' wrote Roman historian Suetonius in 121 AD. 'Because
of it he used to comb forward his scanty locks from the crown
of his head.'[1] That's right, the dictator of the Roman Republic
had a comb over. Caesar's lover, the Egyptian queen Cleopatra,
desperately invented a hair-promoting paste of powdered horse
teeth and deer bone marrow (presumably inspired by the hairiness
of both creatures). It didn't work. To disguise his receding hairline
Caesar routinely donned a laurel wreath, an accessory usually only
worn ceremonially to mark important victories.

Caesar considered baldness a frailty that compromised his
persona of absolute power. Little did he know that two millennia
later, baldness could offer an advantage to Russian men seeking
election. By some cosmic quirk, ever since the balding Nicholas I
became Emperor of Russia in 1825, Russia's leaders have alternated
between being bald and hairy. There are no exceptions. Let's
dive in at the outbreak of the Russian Revolution in 1917. We've
got Lenin, who was bald. Then Stalin, hairy. Khrushchev bald.
Brezhnev, hairy. Andropov, bald. Chernenko, hairy. Gorbachev,
bald. Yeltsin, hairy. Putin, bald. Medvedev, hairy. Then Putin
again, still bald. The 'bald-hairy' phenomenon, as the Russians

call it, started as a joke when it was first noticed in the 1970s but has persisted as an eerie reality.

Caesar didn't even enjoy the silver lining of being credited as the inventor of the comb over. That dubious honour went to American father-son duo Frank and Donald Smith, who in 1977 patented Caesar's comb-over technique as 'a method of styling hair to cover partial baldness using only the hair on a person's head'.[2] US patent 4,022,227 explains how 'the hair styling requires dividing a person's hair into three sections and carefully folding one section over another'. The addition of a laurel wreath is optional.

*

Humans are fairly bald compared to most other mammals. Sea otters, for instance, have more hairs per square centimetre of skin than humans have on their whole scalp. Besides those creepy hairless cats and naked mole rats (if you've not seen one, imagine a bald miniature walrus), it's hard to think of many other mammals with as much exposed skin as us. Humans' relative hairlessness is unique among all primate species. Other primates are draped in luscious locks: orange orangutans, stripy-tailed lemurs, frizzy blonde baboons. Distinctive haircuts and colours even inspired the names of several primate species, like silverback gorillas, cotton-top tamarins (who sport a white mohawk) and capuchin monkeys (who, along with the drink 'cappuccino', were named after their similar colour to the milky brown robes worn by Capuchin monks).

We named our species *Homo sapiens* – 'wise man' – but perhaps we should have gone with *Homo gymnos* – 'naked man' (the word 'gymnasium' is from the Greek for 'naked place', since nude training was once the norm).

Going nude helped our ancestors survive on the savannah. Keeping cool became a priority when we descended from damp forest trees to roam the open grasslands. Hunting under the blazing daytime sun was impossible for anybody insulated by a thick fur coat. But less hairy hominids could venture out during the day to hunt and find food without being incapacitated by heat, because their exposed skin allowed radiant heat loss. Selection pressure also favoured those with increased sweat gland density, which offered evaporative cooling benefits. Sweaty, less hairy bipedal hominids could run longer distances without overheating. Eventually we tamed fire and could fashion clothes to keep our bodies warm at night, negating the need for body fur. And thus, the naked ape evolved.

Technically, humans aren't truly naked. We have the same density of hair follicles as other apes, but many of our hairs are exceptionally fine. What's not fine is their propensity to fall out and cause people significant psychological stress in the process.

*

A hair is a strand of gummed-together dead cells emerging from a tunnel in your skin called a follicle. Follicles cover every square millimetre of your skin except your lips, the palm sides of your hands and the soles of your feet. Over your life each of your five million follicles will grow and shed single hairs in repeated cycles. Scalp follicles, for instance, will nurture about 20 hairs each. After one hair falls out, another grows. Each follicle cycles independently, which prevents en masse balding. If follicles cycled in sync, you'd occasionally wake up bald or without eyebrows when all your follicles entered their 'shed' phase.

Just two per cent of your follicles – about 100,000 of them – are on your scalp. The average varies with hair colour. Brunettes have between 75,000 to 150,000 scalp follicles while blondes have 10 per cent more and redheads 10 per cent fewer.

Your hair is naturally dyed by cells called melanocytes, which produce the pigment melanin. Melanin comes in two varieties: eumelanin (which can be black or brown) and the red-tinged pheomelanin. Despite this limited colour palette, every human hair colour can be produced by some combination of these two pigments. If your melanocytes make lots of inky black eumelanin, you'll have black hair. Hairs weakly dyed with brown eumelanin are blonde; stronger concentrations produce rich chocolate hairs. After you're born, brown eumelanin production can take a while to kick in, which is why platinum-blonde children can grow into brunettes. Strawberry-blonde hairs have low concentrations of both brown eumelanin and pheomelanin. Red hairs, unsurprisingly, contain mostly pheomelanin.

Your genes determine the age at which your melanocytes will start failing to produce melanin, allowing unpigmented grey or white hairs to sprout. Your genes also account for hair colour variation across your body. Multiple genes control the type and amount of melanin in your hair. Follicles at different sites vary in how they express those genes. A man's beard and scalp hair often don't match due to slight differences in pigment ratios. Often there's higher pheomelanin production on the jawline which results in random red beard hairs. Greater eumelanin production in your eyebrow and eyelash follicles accounts for their darker pigmentation.

A hair begins as a bulb of living cells at the base of a follicle. Pluck out a scalp hair and examine its root: the bulb is that swollen blob on the tip. Each of your five million follicles has a tiny muscle (an *arrector pili*; Latin for 'upright hair') attached to it, just above the bulb. The other end of each muscle is buried in the overlying skin. When the muscle tightens it tugs the hair upright to create a 'goosebump'. Blood vessels deliver nutrients to the hair bulb, allowing its cells to divide. Newly born cells are injected with melanin and start filling the follicle tunnel from the base. Constant cell production pushes the older cells sitting on top of them towards the skin's surface. Oily sebum secreted by the follicle's sebaceous gland keeps the follicular tunnel lubricated. Ascending cells are slowly cut off from the bulb's blood supply and start dying. In their death throes they form a sticky protein called keratin. As keratin hardens it entombs the dead cells to form a solid strand. Ongoing cell division down at the hair bulb pushes the hard strand through the follicle until it reaches your skin's surface. You experience the emerging strand of hardened dead cells as your hair growing.

Right now, about 90 per cent of your scalp follicles are in this growth phase of their lifecycle. But hairs don't grow forever. A hair's maximum possible length depends on the duration of its growth phase, which varies according to body site and your genes. Most people's scalp hairs keep growing for two to six years before they fall out. Holders of Guinness's 'world's longest hair' records are genetically equipped with considerably longer growth phases (Chinese woman Xie Quiping has held the record since 2004 when, after 31 years of growth, her hair was 5.627 metres /18.461 feet long). Eyebrow hairs have a growth phase of just two to three months. Try as you might, you'll never succeed in growing eyebrow dreadlocks. Similarly, short growth phases account for why you've never had to trim your eyelashes or forearm hair. Growth speed also varies around your body. Head hair emerges at 0.3 millimetres per day (about a centimetre per month) compared to glacial eyebrow extension at 0.1 millimetre per day.

The remaining 10 per cent of your scalp follicles are in their 'rest phase'. Once a hair's growth phase ends, the hair bulb unplugs from its blood supply and retracts towards your scalp's surface. The detached hair sits in the follicle for about 100 days until your comb's teeth or your vigorously shampooing fingers provide the final parting yank. Between 50 and 100 scalp hairs naturally shed like this every day. The newly vacated follicle will then enter its growth phase again.

You can tell what growth phase a hair is in by what its bulb looks like. If you've got enough to spare, pluck out a few more scalp hairs for bulb examination. A darkly pigmented, chunky bulb is characteristic of a hair in its growth phase. The blood-starved bulb of an imminently falling hair in its rest phase looks like a hard, white node. If you can't see a bulb you've probably snapped the hair off mid-shaft.

*

When you were the size of a strawberry at 10 weeks' gestation you started forming hair follicles. Not hairs yet, just the skin tunnels from which hairs would soon emerge. Follicles formed in a single wave starting in the skin on your brow and finishing at your feet by 22 weeks' gestation. By this point you were coconut-sized, and, like a coconut, were hairy. Newly formed follicles had been at work extruding fine, soft, translucent hairs called *lanugo* (Latin for 'wool'). Before long, a two to three-centimetre (about an inch) fluffy lanugo coat covered your entire body: face, chest, back, everywhere. You eventually shed your woolly coat during your seventh and eighth month *in utero*. What happened to the loose hairs, you ask? You ate them. Your first bowel movement, called meconium, contained the remnants of your foetal fleece.

After birth, your follicles diverged into two populations depending on their location. Some follicles enlarged and started producing thick coloured strands called terminal hairs, like the ones on your scalp, plus your eyelashes and eyebrows. Most follicles stayed puny and spouted short, colourless vellus hairs (Latin for 'fleece'). Look at your earlobe. Those are vellus hairs. Many vellus hairs aren't even visible: they never grow long enough to protrude from the follicle.

Puberty is associated with a surge in steroid hormones called androgens. The two most important androgens are testosterone and dihydrotestosterone, the latter being significantly more potent. Despite *andro* being Greek for 'male', girls also produce small quantities of androgens. Androgens cause things to grow: muscles, bones, vocal cords (see *Voice (loss of)*, page 143), sebaceous glands (see *Acne*, page 281) and follicles. Thick, dark pubic hairs emerge during puberty as androgens transform certain vellus follicles into terminal ones. Follicles all over your body vary in their sensitivity to androgens. Particularly sensitive sites are the genitals and underarms, where even the low androgen levels in girls are enough to convert vellus follicles to terminal ones. Boys' higher androgen levels reach the 'terminal transition' threshold at more locations including the upper lip, lower face, chest, limbs, and back of the hand and fingers.

It seems simple: androgens make follicles grow. But it's men who go bald with age, not women. Surely androgen-depleted women should be the ones losing their hair? And why can bald men still grow luxurious beards?

It's called the 'androgen paradox'. Androgens make beard hairs grow, but scalp hairs shrink. Nobody knows why scalp follicles have this reaction to androgens. It's called a paradox for a reason. We can't explain the androgen paradox, but here's what we do know about how balding happens.

Testosterone reaches hair follicles as it flows through the blood. When testosterone reacts with *5-alpha reductase,* a chemical in hair follicles, it forms that other much stronger androgen dihydrotestosterone (DHT). Facial follicles thrive on DHT, which allows bushy beards to grow. But on the scalp, DHT turns chunky terminal follicles into vellus ones. DHT slashes the growth phases of scalp follicles until they're so brief that the hairs can never grow long enough to become visible. DHT's combined effects progressively 'miniaturise' (that's the legitimate medical term) scalp follicles until you're left with a bald head.

Hair loss progresses in a typical pattern that reflects variations in how sensitive the scalp follicles are to DHT. First to go are the super-sensitive follicles on either side of the hairline, creating an M-shaped widow's peak. A bald spot atop the head soon looms. The spot expands and the hairline recedes until they make a demoralising merger. All that remains is a semicircle of hair stretching ear to ear along the neckline. For unknown reasons, the follicles in that semicircle thrive on DHT just like beard follicles.

These stages of balding are represented visually by the seven-point Hamilton-Norwood scale used by doctors to classify the extent of a man's baldness. We'll meet Dr James Hamilton in a moment; Dr O'Tar Norwood, a pioneer of hair transplants, joined the scale's name when he updated it in 1970. About half of men aged from 40 to 49 show 'moderate to extensive' balding, defined as at least stage 3 on the Hamilton-Norwood scale (a prominently receding hairline, possibly with an emerging bald patch).[3]

A man's genes determine his propensity to hair loss. Some men just happen to have very DHT-sensitive scalp follicles. Other men have high scalp concentrations of *5-alpha reductase* that swamp follicles with DHT. Either way, the outcome after puberty is the same: progressive balding driven by sustained adult-level androgen production. Highly genetically susceptible men start losing their hair soon after puberty and rapidly progress through the Hamilton-Norwood balding stages.

It's baffling and maddening that one hormone can have opposite effects on follicles mere millimetres from each other – balding on the head, flourishing on the face. As a silver lining, the androgen paradox underlies the success of hair transplants as a treatment for baldness. If some DHT-loving follicles are surgically transplanted from your jawline to your scalp, they'll keep on growing. Unlike your bank balance post-op.

*

For millennia, people have noticed that castrated men don't go bald. Greek physician Hippocrates observed that Persian eunuchs guarding the king's harem never went bald. The same could not be said of Hippocrates himself, who tried to regain his vanishing hair with a concoction of horseradish, beetroot, spices, opium and pigeon faeces. It didn't work. Hippocrates concluded that 'hot blood' in virile men like himself caused balding, but castrated men devoid of 'hot blood' kept their hair. Presumably the hot blood singed off the scalp follicles. Greek polymath Aristotle (384-322 BC) had further musings on baldness:

> Men go bald visibly more than any other animal ... no one goes bald before the time of sexual intercourse ... Women do not go bald because their nature is like that of children ... Eunuchs do not become bald because they change into the female condition.[4]

Considering that Aristotle knew nothing about hormones – or gender equality, apparently – those are some spectacularly salient observations. It wouldn't be until 1905 that the word 'hormone' (from the Greek for 'that which sets in motion') would be coined, while testosterone would only be characterised and named in 1935. For years, scientists had suspected the existence of a testicle-based virility-giving substance. For example, in 1889, 72-year-old French neurologist Charles Brown-Sequard injected himself with testicular extracts from guinea pigs and dogs and reported on their rejuvenating effects. 'I had regained at least all the strength I possessed a good many years ago,' he gushed.[5] A trend for 'organotherapy' followed, which involved injecting fluids from animal testicles and other organs in an attempt to prevent aging and treat disease. It didn't work.

A breakthrough in balding research came in 1942. Yale University anatomist Dr James Hamilton (of the balding scale fame) had been investigating 'the relationship of the testes to the status of head hair' among 104 men who had lost their testicles at different life stages.[6] None of the men who had been castrated before puberty went bald. 'Hairs continued to grow not only over the temples, but also along the side of the forehead almost to the lateral edges of the eyebrows.' Men who were castrated later in life, after balding had already started, immediately stopped balding when their testicles were removed. But if any castrated man received androgen replacement injections, he resumed balding.

Hamilton had scientifically proven that androgens cause balding. Finally, we knew the real reason why castrated men (and women) didn't go bald: the lack of androgens (not the lack of hot blood). A man's testicles are his main source of testosterone. Women, and men without testicles, produce only traces of testosterone from their adrenal glands (and ovaries in women). Minimal testosterone means minimal DHT production and thus minimal balding. But women aren't entirely spared from androgen-driven balding. Women who produce excess androgens due to ovarian cysts, tumours or other diseases can suffer balding just like men.

Not all cases of balding can be blamed on androgens. Hair loss can result from autoimmune diseases, where a misguided immune system attacks hair follicles. Balding is also a common side-effect of certain drugs used to treat cancer. Chemotherapeutic drugs kill cells that replicate quickly like tumour cells (which is why chemo works), but also cells lining your mouth (causing ulcers), intestines (causing diarrhoea), and hair bulb cells (causing baldness). Some chemotherapy regimens don't cause significant hair loss, but those that do are toxic to *all* of your hair follicles, not just the ones on your scalp. Eyebrows, eyelashes, pubic hairs and head hair can all be expected to drop out. After chemotherapy your follicles take a while to return to normal hair production. The initial regrowth often has an unusual texture and colour; it may even be grey until your melanocytes kick their pigment production back into gear.

Major physical or psychological stress can abruptly shift your scalp follicles from their multi-year growth phase into their three-month rest phase. I once treated a distraught woman who claimed she had gone bald over the Easter weekend. She provided a plastic bag full of long brunette locks to prove it. When I enquired if some traumatic event had happened about three months ago, she looked at me incredulously. Her son had been killed in a car accident on New Year's Day.

*

Essentially, a hair is just a filament of adherent dead cells hanging off your skin. When it comes to the scalp, humans place enormous emphasis on the length, volume, colour and possession of these strands. Ever since Caesar and Cleopatra, balding has evoked emotions of disgust, pity and mockery. Japanese men with comb overs are jeeringly called 'barcode men' inspired by the linear arrangement of plastered-down black hairs against a pale scalp. Disdain for balding is inherent in the medical term for balding, alopecia, which comes from the Ancient Greek for 'fox-mange', *alōpekía*. Apparently bald people are reminiscent of mite-ridden foxes, who rub off their fur from intolerable itch. But we humans don't actually need hair on our heads. Being bald carries no health risks. The only problem with balding is the social stigma.

SUMMARY: Androgens cause hair follicles on the scalp to shrink and stop growing, resulting in progressive balding. We don't know why. Since men generally have higher androgen levels than women, men go bald with age while women don't.

AND ALSO ...

Fruity language

Testosterone comes from testicles. So does the word 'avocado'. 'Avocado' is from the Nahuatl (Aztecan) word *aguacate* which meant both 'avocado' and 'testicle', given their shared shape and tendency to grow in pairs.

Hair direction

Hairs on your body grow at different angles depending on what direction your foetal skin was being stretched when the follicles formed. From their initial 'straight up' growth direction, your follicles were dragged to face different angles by elongating limbs and growing organs. For example, the sloping angle of your head hairs results from rapid brain expansion stretching the scalp during weeks 10 to 16 of gestation. As your dome-shaped brain grew backwards, follicles in the taut scalp skin were also angled backwards. Grab a mirror and look at the whorl of hair on the back of your head. The middle of that whorl marks the surface point under which maximum brain growth was occurring in utero. Hair patterns can be strikingly abnormal in babies with structural brain problems. If their brain didn't have the usual scalp-stretching growth spurt, their whorl may be missing, and their hair may stick straight out rather than having the usual backwards slope. Uneven brain growth can cause multiple hair whorls, or patches of hair growing against the grain.

Fighting a war on facial hair

Facial hair has a chequered history in the military, being both mandated and prohibited at various times. Moustaches, considered a sign of virility, became compulsory in 1854 for troops in the East India Company's Bombay Army. The British Army soon followed suit. Between 1860 and 1916, British soldiers were disciplined if they tried to shave off their moustache. As per Command No. 1695 of the King's Regulations, passed in 1906: 'The hair of the head will be kept short. The chin and under-lip will be shaved but not the upper lip. Whiskers, if worn, will be of moderate length.' The policy was abandoned in World War I when men complained that their moustaches were endangering their lives by preventing an adequate seal on their gas masks. The abolishment order was signed by General Sir Nevil Macready, who famously despised his mo':

[After signing the order] I dropped into a barber's shop and set the example that evening, as I was only too glad to be rid of the unsightly bristles to which I had for many years been condemned by obedience to regulations.[7]

The Royal Airforce never fell for the 'virility' nonsense and imposed a blanket ban on all facial hair until a policy update on 1 September 2019 which permitted 'neatly-trimmed' beards in an attempt to spur recruitment and foster inclusivity.

The Royal Navy's procedure manual outlines its hair and beard regulations in startling detail, complete with explanatory diagrams. Prohibited facial hair styles include 'handlebar moustaches', 'designer stubble' and 'extended or 'hipster' beards'.[8] Any beard that your Commanding Officer considers 'scrappy' or 'taking an excessive time to grow' (two weeks is the suggested cut-off) may also receive the razor treatment.

ENDNOTES

1   Suetonius. *The Life of Julius Caesar.* Translated by Rolfe, J. C.

2   Smith F. J. *Method of concealing partial baldness.* US Patent 4022227A (1977).

3   Rhodes, T., et al. Prevalence of male pattern hair loss in 18-49 year old men. *Dermatology Surgeon*, 24 (12), 1330-1332 (1998).

4   Aristotle. *On the Generation of Animals.* Translated by Platt, A. Book V, Ch. 3.

5   Brown-Séquard, C. Note on the effects produced on man by subcutaneous injections of a liquid obtained from the testicles of animals. *The Lancet*, 2, 105-107 (1889).

6   Hamilton, J. Male hormone stimulation is prerequisite and an incitant in common baldness. *American Journal of Anatomy*, 71 (3), 451–480 (1942).

7   Macready, N. *Annals of an Active Life, Volume 1.* Hutchinson & Company (1925).

8   Naval Personnel Management. *Chapter 38 Policy and Appearance* (version 10), Edition of BR 3, Volume 1 (2016).

EARACHE

'Last Sunday at 11:30 pm, painter Vincent Van Gogh ... presented himself at brothel number one, asked for a "Rachel" and handed her his ear, telling her "keep this object carefully".'

- Le Forum Républicain, **30 December 1888**

English is full of euphemisms: 'between jobs' is the polite way to describe someone who is unemployed; 'doesn't suffer fools gladly' is code for an impatient jerk; 'eccentric' refers to someone who is crazy, but rich. Vincent Van Gogh, who only sold one painting during his life and died destitute, was considered 'crazy'. Florence Foster Jenkins, however, was an 'eccentric' New York socialite at the turn of the 20th century who fancied herself as an opera singer, despite being tone-deaf. *Life* magazine described her as 'probably the most complete and utter lack of talent ever publicly displayed in Manhattan', and complained that 'listening to her pathetic bleating is something like eavesdropping on a padded cell inmate'.

Jenkins was infected with syphilis at the age of 18. One theory goes that the toxic effects of her pre-penicillin era treatment – mercury and arsenic – may have caused hearing loss due to heavy metal toxicity. Her self-perceived talent may have represented a delusion of grandeur, a typical feature of late-stage syphilis. What's undisputable is Jenkins' defiant claim: '... people may say I can't sing, but no one can ever say I didn't sing.'

Lopping off one's ear for a prostitute, or enduring hours of off-key opera singing are effective methods of achieving an earache. A less melodramatic though certainly more prevalent cause is a middle ear infection.

When you imagine an ear, you're probably picturing the external ear. Those odd folds of skin and cartilage funnel sound waves into your ear canal, a skin and wax-lined tube roughly the length of a small paperclip. Incidentally, in Van Gogh's second language, French, the word for a paperclip is 'trombone' since that's what it looks like. They also call the musical instrument a 'trombone' (context being sufficient to avoid confusion). Your eardrum seals the end of your ear canal.

The eardrum is just a sheet of skin that has received exceptional PR. Some people seem to think that the eardrum is made of some magical material like the woven mane of a unicorn. Hearing of an eardrum 'rupturing' usually evokes images of blood gushing forth from the ear canal. Nope, your eardrum is simply skin. If you poke a hole in it, it'll grow right back, just like a hole in the skin on your kneecap would.

Swimmers commonly get external ear infections, known as swimmer's ear. Submerging your head in a swimming pool floods your ear canal with bacteria. Any abrasions to your ear canal's skin, like microscopic scratches from earphones or cotton tips, provide easy entry for bacteria. I once treated a patient whose external ear infection resulted from a drunken experiment to see how many paperclips he could 'jam down [his] earhole'. He managed six before blood started coming out.

Surfers have their own unimaginatively named ear complaint: 'surfer's ear'. Wave riders' ear canals are regularly blasted with icy water and wind while they hang loose at the line-up. These cold stimuli trigger lumps of bone to grow into the ear canal as an adaptation to protect the eardrum from the cold. The narrowed canal is prone to trapping water and debris – a cesspool for infection. To complete the list of blandly named profession-based ear complaints, add boxer's ear. Your ears' convoluted cartilage creases don't have their own blood supply. The cartilage is kept alive by blood vessels coursing through the skin that's firmly stuck to it. Punches to the ear can burst those blood vessels. The puddle of blood that gathers under the skin separates the cartilage from its life-sustaining skin coating. Unless the clotted collection is cleared, the nutrient-starved cartilage below will die. Also called 'cauliflower ear', the dead withered cartilage results in a disfigured ear.

Behind the eardrum sits an air-filled chamber called the middle ear. It's a pea-sized, bony box lined with skin and spanned by a string of bones (see *Hearing loss*, page 85). The middle ear is quite isolated. Its only connection to the outside world is via a pipe called the eustachian tube* (pronounced 'you-station') which runs from the floor of the middle ear to the back of your throat. *The back of your throat!* This was among the most unsettling facts that I learnt at medical school. Yes, middle ear juices trickle down this anatomical straw, drip into your throat just above and behind your uvula (the dangly bit at the back of your mouth), and then you swallow them. You can't unthink that description, so let's just proceed.

Normally, the eustachian tube's walls are collapsed flat against each other. This stops adventurous throat germs from hitching a ride up the tube into your middle ear. Every time you swallow, you flex a tiny muscle called the *tensor veli palatini* (from the Latin for 'to stretch' and 'the veil of the palate'). When this muscle tightens it draws up your soft palate like a curtain. This action props open your eustachian tube and allows the middle ear to drain.

To hear properly, the pressure on either side of the eardrum must be the same. If your ear canal on one side, and your middle ear on the other are filled with air under different pressures, the

---

* Named by Italian anatomist Antonio Valsalva (1666–1723) in honour of Bartolomeo Eustachi (c. 1513–1574), another Italian anatomist who first described the eustachian tubes.

eardrum won't vibrate normally. Thus, the eustachian tube's second job, besides acting as a sewerage pipe for the middle ear, is to act as a pressure valve. Periodically opening to allow air to travel between the middle ear and outside environment (via your throat) equalises air pressure. That 'pop' you hear when changing elevation is the sound of the pressure in your middle ear equalising with the surrounding atmosphere.

Say you've just lifted off in a hot air balloon. As you ascend, the air pressure around you is decreasing. But the air pressure in your middle ears, being isolated air chambers, is the same as it was at ground level. Your eardrums will start to bulge into your lower-pressure ear canals until – *pop!* – your eustachian tubes allow a tiny bubble of air to escape from each middle ear into your throat. With pressure equalised, your bulging eardrums will return to their usual flat position and resume their normal function.

Until your eustachian tubes do their job, your increasingly stretched eardrums will become increasingly painful. If you're in an ascending plane and your aching ears just won't pop, you can try to coax your eustachian tubes into opening by forcibly yawning, repeatedly swallowing, chewing some gum, or sucking on a lollipop. All of these actions activate your *tensor veli palatini* muscles. By repeatedly raising 'the veil of the palate' you should provide your eustachian tubes with ample opportunity for air pressure equalisation. Italian anatomist Antonio Valsalva, between dissecting cadavers and sampling their bodily juices,* devised his own eponymous manoeuvre to open the eustachian tubes. To perform the Valsalva manoeuvre, close your mouth, pinch your nose, and blow out as if you're inflating a balloon. The air you're trying to blow out should shoot up your eustachian tubes to make your ears 'pop'. If all these methods fail, at least you've got a lollipop to ease the pain.

---

* Valsalva was known to taste the fluids he encountered while performing post-mortems in order to better characterise them: 'Gangrenous pus does not taste good, leaving the tongue tingling unpleasantly for the better part of the day'.

Screaming children on planes with yet-to-equalise middle ears are seldom rational enough to heed advice regarding *tensor veli palatini* activation techniques or to attempt Valsalva manoeuvres. Here, the Politzer manoeuvre may be useful. The technique requires a device akin to a bike pump: a narrow hose attached to a handheld balloon. Insert the hose up one of the toddler's nostrils and, at the moment they stop sobbing to swallow, squeeze the balloon to deliver a puff of air up their nose. If well-timed, the jet of air should blast up their nostril, into the back of their throat and up their eustachian tubes as they naturally open with swallowing.

As the middle ear's sole lifeline for drainage and air pressure equalisation, a working eustachian tube is extremely important. The majority of earaches happen when the eustachian tube becomes blocked.

In children, the eustachian tube is small (like most parts of children). It's prone to becoming obstructed simply because it's so narrow. Another common tube-blocker – in kids and adults – is swelling around its opening in the throat. This swelling can be due to allergies or upper airway infections like colds. Since kids have both smaller eustachian tubes and get lots of colds, they're prone to getting frequent middle ear infections.

Once the eustachian tube is blocked, the middle ear is truly isolated from the outside world. Shed skin and fluid accumulates. Like any stagnant body fluid, it soon becomes infected with bacteria. These bugs multiply, your immune cells join the fight and soon there's a whole crowd of cells, debris and pus (which is just dead white blood cells) within the middle ear. Without the eustachian tube as an exit route, this gunk has nowhere to go. Pressure builds up in your middle ear, stretches your eardrum, and causes ... yep, you guessed it – an earache.

Usually your immune system clears up the infection within a few days. The eustachian tube swelling settles down, it reopens, and pain relief soon follows as the accumulated pus oozes into your throat. Particularly nasty infections can cause the middle ear pressure to skyrocket as it fills with briskly breeding bacteria. If the eustachian tube remains swollen shut the pus will burst through the weakest alternative exit: your eardrum. Usually this provides instant pain relief. Your hearing will drop off in that ear until the eardrum skin (remember, it really is just skin) grows back in a couple of weeks.

Children who get recurrent middle ear infections not only suffer earache, but they can also fall behind at school since they can't hear what their teachers are saying. Sound doesn't travel well through a pus-filled middle ear. Ever-practical otolaryngologists (ear, nose and throat specialists) have a simple solution: make a backup drainage route that will work when the eustachian tube doesn't. In an incredibly simple procedure (no offence, otolaryngologists), the surgeon inserts a tiny plastic tube called a grommet into the eardrum. In the event of a eustachian tube blockage, any middle ear gunk can now drain out the ear canal through the grommet, bypassing the blocked eustachian tube. The grommet will harmlessly fall out onto the kid's pillow after a year or so, buying time for the child's eustachian tube to widen up a bit into a reliable drainage pipe.

Grommets aren't just for eardrums: a grommet is the generic name for a ring that preserves a hole in some material. Eyelets in shoes for threading laces are grommets. Grommets stop the holes in curtain material from fraying as the curtain rod slides through them. Electricians thread delicate cables through rubber grommets in metal sheets. Gromit, the dog in the claymation series *Wallace and Gromit*, was named after these handy rings. Nick Park, the series' creator, had an older brother who worked as an electrician and could often be heard discussing grommets. Nick, after deciding that 'grommet' was a great name for an animated pet, didn't double-check the spelling, and Gromit the clay canine was born (he was originally a cat, but Nick found modelling a dog easier.)

As a domesticated beagle with floppy ears, Gromit would be prone to painful ear infections. A curtain of furry skin draped over the ear canal transforms it into an insulated nook that is ideal for bacterial breeding. Floppy ears also act as a barrier to sound waves reaching the eardrum. Neither of these issues trouble dogs that sport upright ears: pointy ears promote healthy ventilation and more efficiently funnel soundwaves into the ear canal. Droopy ears are, evolutionarily, a terrible idea. Like many terrible ideas, meddling humans are to blame.

When animals become domesticated they acquire certain traits, including the propensity for drooping ears. Charles Darwin's radical 1859 publication, *On The Origin Of Species*, opened with this observation in 'Chapter 1: Variation Under Domestication':

> Not a single domestic animal can be named which has not
> in some country drooping ears; and the view suggested by
> some authors, that the drooping is due to the disuse of the
> muscles of the ear, from the animals not being much alarmed
> by danger, seems probable.[1]

Although Darwin's observation was salient, his support of the drooping from disuse hypothesis was not.

Exactly one century later in 1959, Russian scientist Dmitry Belyaev embarked on an experiment to domesticate the silver fox. Belyaev, like Darwin, had noticed that tame species often had floppy ears. But he noticed that they shared other physical traits too, like smaller faces and blotchy fur. He suspected that these traits were, somehow, genetically linked with tameness. Starting with a skulk of wild foxes, Belyaev would hand-pick the tamest ten per cent of every generation's offspring to parent the next generation. After just six generations Belyaev had produced a handful of foxes that wagged their tails when experimenters approached, licked the humans' hands, could be scooped up and cuddled, and whined when the humans departed. But it wasn't just the behaviour that was similar amongst these tamer foxes. Despite selectively breeding foxes based purely on their temperament, the friendlier foxes had smaller teeth, shrunken skulls and jaws, and white-patched coats. After ten generation the first fox with floppy ears, *Mechta* (Russian for 'dream'), was born.

It turns out that humans can't outfox basic anatomy. As embryos, all vertebrates (animals with spines) have a cluster of cells around their developing spinal cord called the neural crest. As the embryo grows, those neural crest cells migrate and give rise to multiple structures: ear cartilage, pigment cells, skull bones, teeth, and – importantly – the adrenal glands. Those adrenal glands are crucial to orchestrating the fight or flight stress response that drives wild animals to either attack or gallop away from humans. Tame animals, however, have such a dampened fight or flight response that they'll allow us to carry them in shoulder bags.

By only allowing placid foxes to mate, Belyaev was inadvertently selecting for animals with neural crest defects that gave rise to faulty adrenal glands. With each generation, the offspring's increasingly stunted adrenal glands mounted a smaller and smaller stress response to humans.

The other physical features that the foxes shared were just collateral damage from those defective neural crest cells: weak ear cartilage caused floppy ears, errors in pigmentation resulted in white fur patches, and a deformed skull meant a smaller jaw, teeth and brain. Whenever humans domesticate a species, our encouragement of neural crest defects means that these traits invariably emerge. As it happens, humans find floppy ears and patchy fur endearing. Well, until a floppy-eared beagle bites your hand because its earache is making it grumpy.

SUMMARY: Most earaches happen when the middle ear's drainage pipe, the eustachian tube, gets blocked. The isolated middle ear becomes infected and the pressure from accumulating bacteria and pus causes pain.

AND ALSO ...

A Q-tip clue

Americans call cotton buds or tips 'Q-tips', a brand name that has become generic like velcro, xerox and hoover. Rather lamely, the 'Q' stands for 'quality'. Perhaps the clumsy branding was a frantic backpedal from Q-tips' original name upon their 1920s debut: 'Baby Gays'. The Q-tip website doesn't elaborate on this initial name, though it does helpfully explain that 'the word "tips" describes the cotton swab at the end of the stick'.

Poking a cotton bud into your ear canal can graze the skin and allow a painful ear infection to set in. It can also cause a sound-muffling wax impaction (see *Hearing loss*, page 89). But for German authorities in 2009, Q-tips caused more of a headache than an earache.

'The Phantom of Heilbronn', as she was dubbed by the German media, was an alleged master criminal whose crimewave spanned 1993 to 2009. Her DNA was found at over 40 crime scenes in France, Austria and Germany, on items as disparate as a toy gun, cookie crumbs and a syringe of heroin. The Phantom's *modus operandi* was erratic. Between her six murders (including strangling a pensioner and killing a policewoman) she engaged in less serious crimes like school break-ins.

Security cameras often failed to capture her. When she *was* spotted, witnesses said she looked like a man. If alleged accomplices were nabbed, they vehemently denied her existence. A 300,000 euro reward for information leading to her capture went unclaimed. With every lead exhausted, police desperately consulted psychics.

The mystery was finally solved in 2009 by police trying to identify a burnt corpse. Suspecting it was a particular asylum seeker, they swabbed the fingerprints on his historical asylum application to obtain reference DNA. Inexplicably, *his* fingerprints contained *female* DNA. The Phantom of Heilbronn's DNA.

It was subsequently determined that the 'Phantom' was an unidentified female worker in a Bavarian Q-tip factory. Her DNA had contaminated the police's Q-tip collection. Although the cotton swabs were sterilised before use, that process doesn't remove DNA. The humiliating explanation led to a headline in the local *Bild* newspaper justifiably asking 'Are the heads of our Police stuffed with cotton wool?'

Hippocrates the hypocrite

Hippocrates' earache treatment was to lie to his patient:

> If the ear is painful, wrap up some wool around your finger, pour on some warm oil, then place the wool in the palm of your hand and then place it in the ear until the patient believes something has come out. Then deceitfully throw it into the fire.[2]

At least this more practical than obtaining drops made from 'the brain of a lion mixed with oil', the earache cure suggested by Persian physician Muhammad ibn Zakariya al-Razi (854 BC – 925 BC).[3]

ENDNOTES

1 Darwin, C. *On the Origin of Species*, p. 11 (1859).
2 Hippocrates. *Epidemics*, 6.5, 400 BC.
3 Muhammad ibn Zakariya al-Razi. *The Comprehensive Book on Medicine*, c. 925 BC.

HEARING LOSS

What did you say?

In an example of deafening irony, English town crier Keith Jackman was rendered deaf by his own bell. 'Twenty-five years of ringing the bell in my right hand has had an effect on my hearing; I guess it's an occupational hazard,' explained Keith in 2008, then aged 86. 'My hearing started to deteriorate in my right ear about 10 years ago because I ring the bell in my right hand ... My left ear was okay but in the last couple of years that began to deteriorate as well. Now I can't hear hardly anything at all.' His bell was recorded jingling at 118 decibels: as loud as a clap of thunder.

Since a handheld bell can clang with that kind of force, it's perhaps not surprising that London's original 'Big Ben' bell cracked irreparably when its colossal clapper first hit the bowl during testing. Red-faced engineers melted down the fractured bowl, took to the anvil and hammered a stronger Big Ben 2.0. Sixteen white horses, stirrups festooned with ribbons, hauled the new bell across Westminster Bridge in July 1859. But by September the bell had cracked again. Big Ben sat silent for four years until Astronomer Royal Sir George Airy offered a three-part solution: install a lighter clapper, rotate the bowl a quarter turn to present a non-cracked section for striking, and cut a small square where the crack was to stop it spreading. It was a resounding success.

Three of the metal items featured in that Big Ben tale – a hammer, an anvil and a stirrup – inspired the names of the three bones found in your middle ear. The hammer's handle rests against your ear drum, the stirrup's footplate touches your inner ear and the anvil spans the two. Anatomists prefer to speak in Latin, so these bones, collectively called the ossicles, are referred to as the *malleus* (hammer), *incus* (anvil) and *stapes* (stirrup).

When a body part is named after something, the resemblance is usually dubious at best. For example, the point where your trachea (windpipe) forks in two is called the *carina* (Latin for 'keel') after its non-existent resemblance to the underside of a boat. Continuing the nautical theme, two amorphous non boat-shaped bones in your hands and feet are named the *scaphoid* (Greek for 'boat-shaped') and *navicular* (Latin for 'little ship') respectively. Your ossicles are the exception to this anatomical poetic licence: they really do look like the contents of a miniature blacksmith's workshop. But unlike their namesakes, they are feather-light and miniscule. Your stirrup is the smallest bone in your body, weighing six milligrams and measuring barely three millimetres across.

Your ossicles' job is to transmit sound vibrations from your eardrum to your inner ear. Imagine you're standing on Westminster Bridge at noon. The clanging Big Ben vibrates air molecules, producing sound waves that radiate across London. Funnelled into your ear canal, some of the sound waves hit your eardrum, causing it and the hammer behind it, to vibrate. The vibration is transmitted through the ossicles, ending in the stirrup whose footplate slams into the inner ear. Specifically, it precisely fits into a skin-lined hole called the oval window: the entrance to the magical cochlea.

The cochlea really is magical. It's responsible for turning those crude ossicle rattlings into nerve signals that your brain can interpret as a bell striking noon. Cochleas look uncannily like snail shells, hence their name (*cochlea* is Latin for 'snail shell'). Each cochlea – one per ear – is a three centimetre-long (about an inch) tube, coiled up into a disc shape. It's filled with fluid that looks identical to water. To keep the fluid contained, its opening (where the snail's head would poke out) is sealed with skin – the oval window.

When the stirrup's footplate collides with the oval window, it sends a wave of fluid rippling through the cochlea. The cochlea's walls are stubbled with about 16,000 tiny hair cells. They're not actually hairs, but under the microscope they do look rather like stubble. Fluid currents passing through the cochlea bend the hair cells like wheat stalks in the breeze. Along your cochlea's spiral, hair cells are 'tuned' to respond to different pitched sounds.

Sound waves travel with peaks and troughs. Higher-pitched sounds travel at higher frequencies: that is, more waves per second (measured in Hertz, Hz). Deeper-pitched sounds travel as lower frequency waves. Most day-to-day sounds range from about 200 Hz (such as a dripping tap) to 8000 Hz (for example, a chirping bird). Frontline hair cells closest to the oval window are excited by higher-frequency sound waves (made by higher-pitched sounds). The lower-frequency sound waves, generated by booming bass notes, travel deeper into your cochlea to stimulate the innermost hair cells. Your cochleas can perceive frequencies spanning about ten octaves: 20 Hz to 20,000 Hz. Dogs can perceive up to 45,000 Hz. Porpoises max out at 150,000 Hz.[1]

When a hair cell bends, it fires off an electrical impulse to your brain. Use your finger to trace a three-centimetre (about an inch) horizontal line just above the top of your ear. Beneath your scalp and skull, you're tracing over a strip of your brain called the auditory cortex. There's another on the other side of your brain, for processing sound from your other cochlea. This nub of brain receives all of the electrical impulses generated by your bending hair cells. Just like your cochlea's hair cells, the nerve cells in your auditory cortices are arranged in order of the frequencies they detect. Nerve cells at the front of the strip (nearer your face) receive input from hair cells deep in the cochlea's spiral: the ones that respond to low-pitched sounds. Frontline hair cells that respond to high-pitched sounds plug into the back of the auditory cortex.

It's incredible: the nerve cells in your auditory cortex are literally arranged like the keys on a tiny piano.

Brain functional Magnetic Resonance Imaging (fMRI) is an imaging technique used to measure brain activity. When a brain region is active, blood flow to that area increases in response to higher oxygen demand. The fMRI machine detects this surge in blood flow and displays it as a flash of colour superimposed on the image of the grey brain beneath. If you play different musical notes to someone being scanned in an fMRI machine you can see their auditory cortices 'light up' on the machine's display screen according to each note's pitch. Play a low note and you'll see a flash at the front of their cortex near their face. Play a high note and another flash a little further back will appear. Play a scale and you can watch the auditory cortex sequentially light up like the keys on a toy keyboard. All possible thanks to a pair of tiny fluid-filled snail shells on either side of your head. I told you the cochlea was magical.

Although your cochlea works via wizardry, the clunky process for sound waves to reach your cochlea is decidedly low-tech. First there's the flimsy skin eardrum. Then there's the cumbersome chain of weirdly shaped bones that communicates with your cochlea by ramming into its front door: the oval window. Why couldn't sound waves just directly vibrate the oval window? Why bother with eardrums and ossicles? The reason is amplification.

Hair cells first appeared on our fishy ancestors in a thin strip running the length of their body to detect movements in the water. We've long since left the ocean, but our hair cells can still only sense movement in an aquatic environment, necessitating a fluid-filled cochlea. This presents a serious problem: sound waves hitting our ears are traveling through air, but the cochlea only recognises those sound waves when they're travelling through fluid. It takes much more force for a sound wave to travel through fluid, since it's denser than air. Without amplification, airborne sound waves would just bounce off your oval window: they wouldn't hit it with enough force to deform it and generate a fluid ripple within the cochlea.

The ossicles solve this problem by channelling the eardrum's vibrations to a single point – the stirrup's footplate. Your eardrum's surface area is about 65 square millimetres, roughly the same as the hole in a drinking straw. But its teeny surface area is still twenty times greater than the surface area of your stirrup's footplate. Since all the force of sound waves hitting your eardrum is concentrated in an area one twentieth the size, the ossicles amplify incoming sound waves by twenty times. It's a similar force-focussing situation to using a thumb tack: press your thumb against a wall and it obviously won't pass through it but use the same amount of force on a thumb tack and the point of the tack – where your force is concentrated – will pierce the wall. With the extra oomph provided by the ossicles, sound waves pass seamlessly from the air to the cochlea's fluid. From your hair cells' perspective, it's like we never left the ocean.

*

Two main issues result in hearing loss. The first is a mechanical blockage to sound waves reaching the cochlea. The second is a dodgy cochlea. Let's consider these problems in more detail, starting at your earhole and working our way deeper in.

About one in 10,000 babies – more boys than girls – is born without an ear canal: the tunnel just never formed. It usually affects one ear (the right more often, for no good reason). Clearly if there's no canal to conduct sound waves, you'll struggle to hear well. Byzantine surgeon Paulus of Aegina first described this condition, called external auditory canal atresia (Greek for 'lack of perforation'), in the 7th century AD. Paulus devised a gruesome procedure to core out a new ear canal. Later surgeons tweaked his technique by adding a final eye-watering step: jamming hot iron probes into the newly formed ear canal to prevent it from closing.

Assuming that both of your ear canals are present, an earwax blockage is the most likely reason that sound waves aren't reaching your eardrum. Technically called cerumen, earwax is a paste of shed skin cells gummed together by your ear canal skin's oily secretions. Earwax exists to waterproof your ear canal, lubricate your eardrum to keep it pliable, and to trap debris and microbes. Its slight acidity provides further antimicrobial properties.

Skin in your ear canal, like skin all over your body, is constantly sloughing off and being replaced. As new skin cells are produced at the eardrum, they push older skin cells in a radiating pattern towards your earhole. This skin cell conveyor belt chugs along at a rate of about 0.1 millimetre per day: the same speed that your fingernails grow. Migrating skin cells drag wax-trapped debris out of your ear canals at this constant leisurely pace to keep your ears naturally clean. More rapid wax expulsion happens whenever you move your jaw to talk or chew. Jaw movements distort your ear canals and dislodge any hunks of wax stuck to their walls, ready to tumble free the next time you tilt your head.

The quickest way to cause a wax blockage is by using cotton tips in a vain attempt to clean your ears. With each ram in, you shove escaping wax back to the start of the conveyor belt. Flushing the ear with a water-filled syringe can dislodge a stubborn wax impaction. Despite routinely performing this procedure when I worked at a GP clinic, I could never coordinate holding the kidney dish against the patient's neck to catch the expelled wax-specked water. Although my patients ended up saturated and flecked with earwax, at least they could clearly hear my apology.

If you don't have a medical-grade syringe handy to perform the flushing, a child's water pistol can also do the trick. In a 2005 case report, Canadian doctor Donald A. Keegan described the circumstances leading to the discovery of this unusual technique:

> A 45-year-old male complained of a profound reduction in
> his left ear acuity while staying at an island cottage in rural

Ontario. His hearing loss was reducing his ability to hear his newborn son cry in the middle of the night, requiring his wife to carry out all late-night childcare. As a result, correction of the problem was considered urgent.[2]

But alas, wrote Keegan, 'Neither a formal ear syringe, nor a syringe of any kind was available on the island.' He continued:

Verbal consent (covering risks and benefits) was obtained from the patient. He then changed into swimming shorts, located himself on an ideal location on the deck and held a Tupperware container (product number 1611-16) to the side of his neck, in lieu of a kidney basin. The Super Soaker Max-D 5000 [a high-powered water pistol] was filled with body-temperature water and then mildly pressurised using the blue hand-pump. The trigger was depressed, releasing a gentle, narrow jet of water ... Midway through the second load's stream, wax particles began to run out of the ear. Just after starting the third load, a large plug of wax burst forth from the patient's ear. The three generations of family members present took turns admiring (or recoiling from) the specimen. The patient exclaimed in joy, 'I can hear again!' ... We feel that prospective randomised trials are warranted to evaluate the utility of the Super Soaker Max-D 5000 in clinical settings.

Besides earwax, sound waves can be stymied en route to the eardrum by bony growths in the ear canal (particularly in surfers), a ruptured eardrum, or a fluid-filled middle ear (see *Earache*, page 74).

But if you still can't hear despite sound waves making it to your cochlea's fluid, it's your cochlea that's the culprit.

Your cochlea's hair cells endure substantial buffeting over your lifetime. Consider the number of times each one swishes about daily, let alone after decades of exposure to music, traffic noise, lawnmowers and day-to-day conversations and clatter.

You're born with a quota of hair cells; you don't sprout new ones and dead ones can't be replaced. As hair cells age, they become brittle, less responsive to stimulation, and generate poorer-quality signals for your brain to decipher. Aging is inevitably associated with some degree of hearing loss due to hair cell deterioration, a condition called *presbycusis* (Greek for 'old man hearing'). About half of those aged over 75 have some degree of hearing loss.

Hair cells that respond to high-pitched sounds (the ones right up the front of the cochlea's spiral) are the first to deteriorate with age. Welsh inventor Howard Stapleton capitalised on this fact with his 2005 invention 'The Mosquito'. This irritating high-pitched alarm squeals at 17,400 Hz: a frequency only audible to people under the age of 25. Placed outside train stations and shops, The Mosquito's piercing sound deters loitering youths, yet goes unnoticed by law-abiding adults. 'It's very difficult to shoplift when you have your fingers in your ears,' Stapleton reasoned.

Here's a typical story of a man with presbycusis. First, he'll insist that women and children, whose voices are inherently higher pitched, 'aren't speaking clearly'. Next, consonant sounds like 'f', 's' and 'th' will drop off his hearing radar because they're higher pitched than vowel sounds. This often manifests as the 'cocktail party effect'. When distracted by ambient noise, the cochlea relies on higher-pitched sounds like consonants to focus its attention. Our man with presbycusis might chastise 'mumbling' waiters because 'beef soup' just sounds like 'ee oo' amid the din of other diners; without competing noise he'd hear the waiter fine. But with time and further frequency loss, even one-on-one conversations in quiet environments become difficult.

Unfortunately, age-related hearing loss can't be prevented, but you can slow your hair cells' inevitable decline by protecting them from loud noises. Have you ever suffered tinnitus – ringing ears – after a concert? If so, you've bashed up your hair cells.

Loud noises generate fluid tsunamis in your cochlea that can physically flatten the hair cells. Usually, healthy hair cells briefly bend over with a fluid ripple, shoot off a message to the brain, then stand up again and remain electrically silent. But a collapsed hair cell, since it's permanently keeled over, sends your brain a constant electrical impulse. Your befuddled brain acts on the information it's receiving: if the electrical impulse hasn't stopped, that means the noise hasn't stopped. People can experience the persistent noise of tinnitus as ringing, hissing, buzzing or even chirping. The pitch of the sound depends on the location of the flattened hair cell along the cochlea's coil.

If a hair cell isn't too badly damaged it can pick itself back up, thus stopping the ringing. But the healing process isn't flawless: too many loud exposures can result in permanent noise-induced hearing loss and tinnitus.

How loud is too loud? To answer that we need to recap some physics. A sound's volume depends on its 'sound pressure level', measured in decibels; essentially, what is the change in air pressure caused by those sound waves? 'Decibel' comes from *deci* (one tenth) and the surname of the scale's developer, Alexander Graham Bell, the Scottish engineer credited with inventing the telephone. The decibel scale is logarithmic: every increase in 10 dB is equal to a 10-fold increase in the sound pressure level. Bell defined 0 dB as 'near silence': the quietest sound a human ear can detect. Normal breathing, at 10 dB, generates a sound pressure level 10 times more powerful than near silence.

With that in mind, let's return to the question: how loud is too loud? Prolonged exposure to sounds above 85 dB – typical lawnmower level – will start to damage your hair cells. Hearing loss usually occurs after fifteen minutes of exposure to 100 dB (like a jackhammer) and just five minutes at 110 dB (such as the noise produced by a riveting machine). Sounds at 120 dB feel genuinely painful, as though a chainsaw is chopping off your ear. A chainsaw does actually run at 120 dB, which is why professional tree loppers always wear ear protection. Things get ugly at decibel readings beyond this: think immediate and permanent hearing damage. A sporting rifle fired one metre (three feet) away from your ears (140 dB) will kill both ducks and hair cells. You'll struggle to see a roaring jet engine (150 dB) due to eyeball vibration. And you certainly won't hear it: 150 dB is the point when your eardrums will burst. The loudest possible sound pressure level is 194 dB. Beyond this the sound wave becomes a shock wave; it's no longer passing *through* air, it's *pushing* air.

Hollywood is the home of noise-induced hearing loss. Bruce Willis's left cochlea's hair cells died, hard, while filming the 1988 thriller *Die Hard*. During his anti-terrorist escapades Bruce finds himself under a table firing a Beretta 92 semi-automatic pistol. The blasts from shooting over 15 extra-loud blanks about 30 centimetres (12 inches) away from his left ear (in a confined space, without hearing protection) rendered him two-thirds deaf in that ear. Some 20 years earlier, in 1967, *Star Trek*'s Captain Kirk and his sidekick Spock (William Shatner and Leonard Nimoy respectively) suffered noise-induced hearing loss following an on-set accident. While filming the episode, *Arena* (which is an anagram of 'an ear', coincidentally), the pair were standing over a pan of explosives that detonated with unexpected exuberance. Ears ringing, still in their *Star Trek* garb, the pair were rushed to an audiologist. After being reassured that Spock's pointed ears were a pre-accident pathology, both men were found to have suffered hearing loss. Due to their orientation to the explosion, Nimoy suffered noise-induced hearing loss in his right ear, Shatner in his left.

Mother Nature can generate far louder sounds than anything Hollywood pyrotechnicians can. On 27 August 1883, the Earth made the loudest sound ever recorded. The volcano island of Krakatau, 160 kilometres (100 miles) west of Jakarta, had just erupted. It's hard to comprehend quite how powerful this eruption was. The blast waves reverberated around the globe four times. People 4800 kilometres (almost 3000 miles) away in Alice Springs, in central

Australia, heard the roar. Red hot material covered an area the size of France. A riot broke out in a prison over 1800 kilometres (1100 miles) away when the explosions were mistaken for a shell attack on the facility. In his ship 60 kilometres (37 miles) from Krakatau, the petrified captain of the British ship *Norham Castle* logged:

> So violent are the explosions that the eardrums of over half my crew have been shattered. My last thoughts are with my dear wife. I am convinced that the Day of Judgement has come.

He was wrong about the end of the world, but he was probably right about the eardrum damage: the pressure reading 160 kilometres (100 miles) from Krakatau (100 kilometres/62 miles further away from the blast than his ship) registered 172 dB.

Avoiding loud sounds isn't just good for your ears, it's good for your sanity. Loud sounds can have adverse psychiatric effects. According to a 1970 Columbia Law Review paper on noise pollution '... prolonged exposure to excessive noise has made rats lose their fertility, turn homosexual, and eat their young.'[3] Such pronounced effects aren't seen in humans, but loud sounds have been used as torture.

As Cold War tensions rose in late 1981, guerrillas from the far-left Red Brigade group held US General James Lee Dozier hostage for 42 days in Padua, northern Italy. 'They put earphones on me and played hard rock music all day long ... do you have any idea what hard rock music can do to a person?' Besides the psychological damage, it also left him permanently hearing impaired. 'I'd argue with the guards, and they'd turn the volume down. Finally, they changed to Gershwin tapes. At least the music was better.'

SUMMARY: Hearing requires sound waves to vibrate your eardrum and ossicles, then physically swoosh hair cells in your cochlea. Hearing loss can result from things that block the sound waves from reaching your cochlea, or damage to the cochlea's hair cells.

AND ALSO ...

Read my lips

People with advanced hearing loss rely heavily on lip-reading, but you'd be surprised how much you do too. When you're speaking to someone, you're receiving two simultaneous sensory inputs: audio (sound waves, via your ears) and visual (light, via your retina). Your brain has to coordinate the two to make sense of them. If the inputs are contradictory, your brain can get creative. Pretend you're sitting in front of a TV screen. A video of a woman saying 'ba ba ba' is shown and you are asked what you hear. 'Ba ba ba', you'll say. Next comes a video of the woman saying 'ga ga ga', but the sound is muted, and the 'ba ba ba' audio from the first video is secretly dubbed instead. When asked what you hear, you'll almost certainly reply 'da da da'. Despite hearing the identical audio – 'ba ba ba' – the contradictory lip movement will baffle your brain into 'hearing' a completely new third sound. Called the McGurk effect, it was first described in a 1976 paper 'Hearing Lips and Seeing Voices' by developmental psychologist Harry McGurk.[4]

A particularly cruel prank

It is possible to be completely deaf, despite having perfectly functional ears and cochleas. A handful of people have been unlucky enough to damage both of their auditory cortices, usually due to stroke or trauma. Their intact cochleas still generate electrical impulses, but these people's damaged brains can't interpret these signals as sound. With one fascinating exception: if you popped a balloon behind them, they'd leap around in fright. While their brain's usual sound processing system is shot, their brainstem can still produce a reflex 'jump' in response to loud sounds detected by the cochlea.

A plug for the wonders of whales

Baleen whales have permanent earwax plugs in their ears. Counterintuitively, these long wads of wax might *improve* their hearing. Since earwax and seawater have a similar density, it's thought that the wax plug helps transmit sound waves from the water to their inner ear. The plug also has another use: it informs scientists of the whale's age. Baleen whales constantly produce earwax, the colour of which depends on their diet at that time. Lighter yellow wax layers have a higher fat content: these layers are deposited during the months when the whale gorges on krill. Less fatty darker wax layers deposit during fasting periods when the whale is migrating. Just like a tree trunk, you can count the rings in a cross section of whale earwax to determine how old it is. A dead blue whale in 2007 provided researchers with a 25-centimetre-long, three-centimetre-wide (10-by-one-inch) plug of wax that one scientist compared to 'a roughed-up candle'.

Blue whales' migration patterns mean that their dietary fat intake – and thus wax stripe colours – alternate every six months. Researchers totted up the rings to glean the whale's age: 24 layers, hence 12 years of age. But this off-putting candle provided more than just a history of that whale's birthdays. Chemical analysis of each layer provided a six-month time capsule of the levels of pollution and mercury in the whale's habitat.

Inventive solutions to hearing loss

At the age of 12, 20 years before he would invent the light bulb, Thomas Edison's hearing began to decline. 'Earache came first,' he recalled, 'then a little deafness, and this deafness increased until at the theatre I could hear only a few words now and then'.[5] Edison attributed his deafness to an incident that occurred when he was 12:

I was trying to climb into the freight car with both arms full of heavy bundles of papers. I ran after it and caught the rear step, hardly able to lift myself. A trainman reached over and grabbed me by the ears and lifted me...I felt something snap inside my head and the deafness started from that time and has progressed ever since.[6]

Instead, Edison's hearing loss probably stemmed from recurrent untreated middle ear infections which eroded his ossicles. Edison considered his deafness an advantage: 'It saves me from many interruptions and much nerve strain'.[7] Were he not hearing impaired, he may never have invented the phonograph:

[Being deaf] has taught me not to rely on my own hearing for judgment. Consequently, I have made recording instruments more delicate than human ears, showing beyond question whether a singer sings in tune, whether a voice has a tremolo, or whether any false notes or sounds are present.[7]

Ever the inventor, Edison devised a novel technique to maximise his hearing: biting the source of the noise. Edison's grand piano and personal phonograph are covered in tooth marks. By clamping down on the wood, the sound vibrations could reach his cochleas via his teeth and jaw bone, bypassing his damaged ossicles.

A deafness 'cure' emerged in the 1920s that was even more creative than anything Edison dreamt up: 'deaf flights'. The aim was to shock deaf people's ears into working again via terrifying aerial acrobatics. Some patients willingly submitted. Others were lured onto planes by their doctor's insistence that the high altitude was somehow good for the ears (they argued that the 'surprise' factor of a sudden nosedive maximised the 'beneficial' ear shock). Doctors prescribed deaf flights and pilots willingly performed them. On his 1925 business card, a young Charles Lindbergh, yet to perform his solo transatlantic flight, listed deaf flights among his services. Suffice it to say that intense fear, evoked by high altitude loop-the-loops or otherwise, does not cure deafness. Nevertheless, anecdotal reports of miracle cures sustained the fad until the late 1920s, despite several deaths from stunts gone wrong. By 1930 it became hard to justify the treatment after the *Journal of the American Medical Association* derided deaf flights as 'usually futile and often fatal'.

Come again?

A misheard phrase is called a mondegreen. Writer Sylvia Wright coined the term in reference to her childhood mishearing of the lyrics in a Scottish ballad: instead of 'and laid him on the green' she heard 'and Lady Mondegreen'. Famous mondegreens include lyrics from *Bon Jovi*: 'It doesn't matter if we make it or not' misheard as 'if we're naked or not' and *Creedence Clearwater Revival*: 'There's a bad moon on the rise', misheard as 'bathroom on the right'.

In the 1960s, the FBI investigated rock group *The Kingsmen* over supposedly obscene lyrics in their rendition of 'Louie Louie'. The actual lyrics were: 'Ah, on that ship; I dream she there; I smell the rose; Ah, in her hair'. The alleged lyrics? 'And on that chair; I lay her there; I felt my boner; In her hair'. Ultimately, the FBI concluded 'because the lyrics of the recording ... could not be definitely determined in the laboratory examination, it was not possible to determine whether this recording is obscene'. They were right, the recording's sound quality was abysmal. What ended up being released was a take that the band thought was a rehearsal.

Lead singer Jack Ely's diction was stymied by dental braces and being forced to sing shouting up into a microphone fixed centrally towards the roof. Despite the group's innocence, 'the FBI guys came to our shows, and they'd stand next to the speakers to see if we were singing anything off-colour'. I hope the agents were wearing ear protection.

ENDNOTES

1 Fay, R. R. *Hearing in Vertebrates: a Psychophysics Databook*. Hill-Fay Associates, Winnetka IL. (1988).
2 Keegan D. A. & Bannister S. L. A novel method for the removal of ear cerumen. *Canadian Medical Association Journal*, 173 (12), 1496–1497 (2005).
3 Hilderbrand, J. Noise Pollution: An Introduction To The Problem And An Outline For Future Legal Research. *Columbia Law Review*, 70, 652 (1970).
4 McGurk, H. & Macdonald, J. Hearing lips and seeing voices. *Nature*, 264 (5588), 746–748 (1976).
5 Markel, H. *Literatim: Essays at the Intersections of Medicine and Culture*. Oxford University Press (2019).
6 Plunkett M. J. *Edison: A Biography*. Lake Press (2019).
7 Samuels, D. W. Edison's Ghost. *Music & Politics*, 10 (2) (2016).

NOSEBLEEDS

**A relentlessly runny nose is distressing,
particularly when what's running is blood.**

Military surgeons don't treat many nosebleeds. Generally, their time is occupied with more pressing matters, like extracting shards of shrapnel from blast wounds or reattaching limbs. A soldier would likely be laughed out of the medical tent if they sought help for something as pedestrian as a nosebleed. But in July 1800, private William Stannion had a really bad nosebleed. Even military surgeon John Hennen was impressed by the torrents of blood issuing from poor Stannion's nose. Upon discovering the 'singular cause' for his plight, Hennen felt compelled to publish a case report, titled: *Mr Hennen's Case of Profuse Epistaxis*:

> William Stannion, a private of the regiment, aged 25, was
> seized in the month of July, 1800, with violent pain in his
> forehead … it was not constant, but when it did occur, which
> was generally at night, it usually lasted for three or four hours
> and was attended with violent haemorrhage from the nose.[1]

Hennen tried packing Stannion's right nostril with lint, but the blood just flowed through it 'with most violence' ('violent' seems to be Hennen's go-to adjective). Efforts to reduce 'congestion of blood in the head', like dunking his head in cold water and remaining in the shade, were similarly ineffective. After four days of intermittent haemorrhage, Hennen decided to squirt some cooled water up Stannion's nose:

> In a few minutes after its use, [Stannion] felt something moving violently in the cavity of the nose, which gave him exquisite pain, and shortly after a substance resembling a clot of blood was discharged; he immediately uttered an exclamation of joy, saying he was relieved from most intense torture, and the haemorrhage ceased altogether in about an hour. I, in the meantime, was occupied in examining the substance discharged, which, to my astonishment ... proved to be a leech, enveloped in coagulated blood. It was of the common size, and its motions were lively. I washed off the gore, and applied it on the hand of one of the hospital attendants; it readily fastened ...

Hennen was stumped as to the leech's origin. Stannion's barracks were over 15 kilometres (nine miles) from any 'fresh water, lake, or stream'. Regardless, Stannion rapidly recovered and remained in good health.

Epistaxis, as used in the title of Hennen's thesis, is the medical term for a nosebleed, from the Greek *epi* (upon) and *stazein* (to drip). But as you'd know if you've had a nosebleed, the experience tends to involve more gushing than dripping – and that's without a blood-sucking parasitic worm nestled up one of your nostrils.

*

Your nose has two main jobs: letting you smell, and letting you breathe. Assuming there's no leech obstruction, inhaled air flows through your nostrils and heads down your trachea. Just behind your breastbone, at about the level of your armpits, your trachea forks into two tubes called bronchi. You've got a left and right bronchus: one heading into each lung. Within each lung each bronchus forks, then both of those tubes fork, then all four of *those* tubes fork (I'll spare you the forking details: there are 23 divisions per lung, on average) to form a convoluted tree of increasingly narrow tubes. The final tubes, less than one millimetre across, open out into grape-like clusters of tiny air sacs called alveoli. In one cubic millimetre of lung tissue you'll find about 170 alveoli. Their walls are just one cell thick: thin enough for gases to move across them.

Breathe in through your nose. Air is inflating the tree of tubes within both your lungs and swirling into your alveoli, which are coated with a film of fluid. The oxygen in your breath dissolves in this fluid while passing across the alveolar wall. It's dumped directly into one of the blood vessels clamped like ivy to the outside of the alveolar cluster. Red blood cells flowing in the vessel snaffle up the oxygen molecules. Inside the red blood cell, oxygen sticks to the iron cores of haemoglobin molecules to hitch a ride around your body. Congratulations! You've just oxygenated some of your blood. Now breathe out.

In the next 24 hours your nose will deliver about another 19,999 breaths to your alveoli. Well, either your nose or your mouth will. Humans have the option of nose or mouth breathing since both holes connect to our trachea. Mouth breathing is useful if you've got a cold, or if you need to rapidly inhale large volumes of air when exercising. But the downside of our mouth being connected to our trachea is that it makes us prone to choking if food goes down the wrong way. Evolution has largely solved this issue with a trapdoor system. Your voice box, at the top of your trachea, is capped with a flap of gristle called the epiglottis. Right now, your epiglottis is sitting in an upright position, leaving your trachea open for air (via either your nose or mouth) to flow in and out of your lungs. When you swallow, your epiglottis momentarily snaps forwards to seal your airway, rerouting saliva and food backwards into your oesophagus. Finish swallowing and it flips back up. If the trapdoor system fails and food accidentally enters your airway, you rely on coughing to eject it (see *Cough*, page 168).

Some species don't have the option of breathing through their mouth. These so-called obligate nasal breathers include horses, rabbits, rodents like mice and rats, camels, llamas and alpacas. Watch some footage of a racehorse galloping across the finishing line and focus on its muzzle. Its nostrils will be flaring wildly to suck in air, but its lips will be clamped shut. Unlike human sprinters, gasping for air isn't an option for horses (hence their prodigious nostrils).

Despite seeming like a handicap, mandatory nose breathing is a useful adaptation in species that are frequently preyed upon. Since all air must pass through their nose, the faint whiff of a predator will never go undetected. It's the position of their epiglottis that renders nose-only breathers physically unable to breathe via their mouth. At rest, your epiglottis just points upwards: it doesn't seal anything. A rabbit's epiglottis, however, rests against the back of its tongue, sealing off the bunny's mouth from both the trachea and oesophagus below. Upon swallowing, its epiglottis momentarily flops open to let the dandelion down, then returns to its resting position blocking the back of the bunny's mouth. Mouth-breathed air physically can't reach a rabbit's trachea. On the plus side, if there's a fox skulking nearby, the bunny's ever-twitching nose won't miss its scent.

For animals that can do it, mouth breathing is really just a backup for when their nose is blocked. Obligate mouth breathers don't exist in nature. In fact, when you were born you were an obligate nasal breather just like a horse. Nasal breathing is an innate ability; mouth breathing only begins to emerge in humans around four months of age as a learned work-around to a blocked nose. Before that age, infants with stuffed-up noses can seriously struggle to breathe. However, a rather cruel 1985 study showed that newborns *can* be forced into early mouth breathing.[2] Researchers somehow convinced 19 mothers to offer up their newborns, aged between one and 230 days of age, for the experiment. One researcher held the infant's nostrils shut while another started a stopwatch. All the baby's mouths eventually gasped open for air. But it took up to 32 seconds of struggling plus significant oxygen desaturation before their lips would finally part.

Nasal breathing has several advantages over mouth breathing. Nostrils aren't just passive air holes. Sticky mucous-covered nose hairs trap inhaled microbes and dust particles, keeping your lungs infection-free and clean. Scents inhaled through the nostrils can alert you to danger (such as leaking gas) and influence social behaviour (like deter a man from proposing to bad-breathed Edna [see *Bad breath*, page 116]).

Perhaps most importantly, nasal breathing humidifies the air you breathe. Humidity refers to air's water vapour content. Room air has about 50 per cent humidity. By the time it's swirled through your warm, wet nostrils it's reached 85 per cent humidity. Air absorbs further moisture from the back of your throat to become fully saturated (100 per cent humidity) by the time it enters your lungs. This is crucial: your lungs *must* remain moist. Remember that oxygen has to dissolve in the fluid lining your alveoli to cross their walls and enter your bloodstream. Oxygen can't move across dry alveolar walls.

In his startling 1877 article *Shut your Mouth and Save your Life*, Dr James Patterson Cassells derides the 'evil consequences' and 'incalculable dangers' of mouth breathing.[3] He foreshadows a future in which there are 'dull-brained, badly-formed, and imperfectly developed mouth-breathing creatures peopling a province or even a country'.

Cassells was being a tad melodramatic, but he's correct in saying that the mouth isn't designed for air humidification. It can't compete with your nose's thick mucous and cosy crevices. Dry air blowing through your mouth will rapidly evaporate your saliva. A dehydrated mouth not only stinks, but as Cassells points out: 'the act of respiration is at last disagreeable and may even become painful'. What's more, those who 'breathe the purest air through a foul cavern' bypass nasal filtration, allowing microbes and dust straight into their lungs.

Your nose's large internal surface area makes it a particularly efficient humidifier. Despite not being able to reach a finger up there, your nasal cavities extend all the way up to between your eyebrows. Insert a tissue-covered finger up one nostril. You'll hit an obstruction about two centimetres (just under an inch) in. That's your inferior turbinate, the lowest of three bony shelves that jut into each nasal cavity. Turbinates increase each nostril's surface area, maximising the volume of air that comes in contact with its steamy lining. Your nasal septum – the wall of cartilage dividing your nasal cavity in half to make two nostrils – provides further humidifying real estate. All up, your nostrils' combined surface area is about the same as three playing cards.

Four pairs of air-filled bony cavities called sinuses extend from your nasal cavity. Their exact biological role is debated, but a few ideas have been put forward. Slow air turnover within the sinuses acts as a warm reservoir to assist the nose with humidification. Hollow sinuses lighten your skull and decrease the load on your neck. Sinuses also increase the resonance of your voice (see *Voice (loss of)*, 143) and act as a crumple zone if you faceplant into something solid. Although their function may be controversial, what's undisputed is the significant facial pain that results from blocked, infected sinuses.

Nasal humidification relies on wet and hot nostrils. Viscous, readily replenished mucous provides the moisture. The heat radiates from arteries running along either side of your nasal septum. Five arteries, in fact, per side. To put this in perspective, your gallbladder receives blood from one artery, your heart from two, your brain four, but each side of your nasal septum gets five. This arterial quintet runs a daringly superficial course, barely covered by a mucous membrane. Their shallow position maximises the heat radiating off them into your nostrils. But it also maximises their vulnerability to being damaged and squirting blood everywhere.

There's a little area on either side of your nasal septum where all five arteries meet, called Little's area. Ninety per cent of nosebleeds start here. New York surgeon James Lawrence Little first described the treacherous area in a series of cases published in 1879.[4] Put another tissue-covered finger up one of your nostrils and touch the septum about two centimetres (under an inch) in. That's Little's area. You've got another little Little's area up your other nostril. The five arteries don't just course through Little's area, they all link up there to form one hot, pulsating plexus. Kiesselbach's plexus, we call it, after German otolaryngologist Wilhelm Kiesselbach, who published a second paper on the bleeding hotspot five years after Little.[5] Since they're all connected, if one artery starts bleeding then blood from the other four will join the stream. Hence the epistaxis experience being one of gushing rather than dripping.

Nosebleed incidence peaks in winter, when the low humidity air dries out your nostrils and makes them prone to splitting and bleeding. You're at higher risk of a heavier nosebleed if your blood doesn't clot properly (due to medication, or various bleeding disorders, for example) or if you have high blood pressure (in this case, think fire hose rather than garden hose).

The leading cause of nosebleeds is trauma. Getting punched in the face will do it, but usually the trauma is self-inflicted: nose-picking. Fingernails are sharp; the lining covering Kiesselbach's plexus is thin. Even notoriously dim-witted Ralph Wiggins of *The Simpsons* could grasp the concept: 'the doctor said I wouldn't have so many nosebleeds if I kept my finger outta there'. Toddlers who shove their finger, their sister's finger, their toothbrush, or their Barbie's leg up their nose (all real examples I've encountered) are bound to split open Kiesselbach's plexus en route. Less experimentative adults tend to get nosebleeds when they have a cold due to enthusiastic blowing plus regular tissue friction. Mysteriously, 80 to 90 per cent of nosebleeds happen out of the blue, invariably at inopportune moments (though an opportune moment for a nosebleed is difficult to nominate).

*

'Lean forward ... no, back! Pinch the tip of your nose – or is it the bridge of your nose? Push on your upper lip!' Unsolicited advice is irksome at the best of times, let alone when you're in a public place and your face won't stop leaking blood everywhere. Let's put the record straight: if you get a nosebleed, ignore nearby good Samaritans and do the following:

First, lean forwards. This protects your clothing. It also stops blood from running down your throat which you might otherwise choke on or swallow. Your guts tend to react to swallowed blood by vomiting, which is an additional discomfort you really don't need. Now, pinch both of your nostrils tightly against your nasal septum. You're trying to physically prevent blood from streaming out of Kiesselbach's plexus sitting in Little's area. You know where Little's area is because I made you touch it. Pinch there. Don't pinch up higher. And for heaven's sake don't squeeze the bony bridge of your nose between your eyes. Even if you were strong enough to crush your nasal bones together all you'd achieve is more bleeding from a broken nose. If you can coordinate a hunchbacked stagger towards a freezer, get an ice pack and hold it over the bridge of your nose. Like all liquids, cold blood flows more slowly.

Keep pinching and icing for ten minutes. Yes, ten minutes. This ensures that your blood has had enough time to form a solid clot to stem further flow. Don't pinch for 30 seconds intervals and release to check if you're still bleeding. You will be. And whatever clot had started to form will have just spattered onto the floor.

If the bleeding won't stop despite these measures, call an ambulance. Occasionally nosebleeds stem from arteries at the back of your nose, rather than from Kiesselbach's plexus at the front. If this is the case, the nose-pinching technique is useless. The arteries at the back of your nose are far beyond your reach. You need a doctor. Preferably a doctor with a lubricated balloon on the end of a stick which, when poked deep into a nostril and inflated, provides the required compression. Other emergency techniques include shoving what are essentially expensive tampons up your nostrils or wheeling you to the operating theatre to cauterise (burn closed) the squirting vessel.

Nosebleeds need not be a big deal if you just remember to lean forward and pinch. But if that doesn't work and the emergency doctors are stumped too, perhaps check if there's a leech up there.

SUMMARY: Your nasal septum is laced on both sides with shallow arteries to humidify inhaled air. If they start bleeding, lean forward and tightly pinch your nostrils for ten minutes. And stop picking your nose.

AND ALSO ...

The risks of cocaine are not to be snorted at

Cocaine causes blood vessels to constrict. In the hospital setting, cocaine-impregnated gauze can be pressed over Kiesselbach's plexus to tighten the arteries and stop a nosebleed. Outside the medical setting, regularly snorting cocaine can permanently shrivel up Kiesselbach's plexus. On the plus side – fewer nose bleeds. On the significant downside – your nasal septum can erode.

Being cartilage, your nasal septum has no blood vessels within it. It's kept alive by oxygen and nutrients diffusing from blood vessels running over it. If those vessels dry up, your septum will die from ischaemic necrosis (tissue death due lack of oxygen). As patches of septum die, small perforations form before eventually the entire septum can cave in.

A death he bloody deserved

Attila the Hun was the blood-thirsty military leader of the Hunnic Empire from 434 to 453 AD. Under Attila's command the Huns pillaged and ransacked their way across Europe. The Huns quickly gained a reputation as barbaric savages. Their expert horsemanship and ruthless brutality saw them decimate cities throughout the Roman Empire and earned Attila the moniker 'the scourge of God'.

Against all the odds, Attila didn't meet his death in battle. He wasn't beheaded or trampled upon or impaled by an arrow. He died from a nosebleed.

The night before his death Attila married Ildico, the last of his many wives. He'd managed to find a window in his calendar between massacres for the wedding, during which he drank and ate heavily. The next morning Attila didn't emerge from his bedroom. His guards nervously tapped on his door: no answer. Increasingly frantic banging culminated in their breaking down the door to discover Attila lying dead in his bed with Ildico weeping inconsolably beside him. Dried blood had formed a crust around Attila's nose and lips. The invincible Attila had suffered a nosebleed overnight but, being too plastered to splutter awake, had choked on the blood and died. Or, put more poetically by Gothic historian Jordanes in 551 AD:

> [Attila] had given himself up to excessive joy at his wedding, and as he lay on his back, heavy with wine and sleep, a rush of superfluous blood, which would ordinarily have flowed from his nose, streamed in deadly course down his throat and killed him, since it was hindered in the usual passages.[6]

ENDNOTES

1   Hennen, J. Mr. Hennen's Case of Profuse Epistaxis. *Medical Physiology Journal*, 11 (64), 549-550 (1804).

2   Rodenstein, D. et al. Infants are not obligatory nasal breathers. *American Review of Respiratory Diseases*, 131 (3), 343-7 (1985).

3   Cassells, J. P. 'Shut Your Mouth and Save Your Life': Being Remarks on Mouth-Breathing, and Some of Its Consequences, Especially to the Apparatus of Hearing: A Contribution to the Ætiology of Ear-Disease. *Edinburgh Medical Journal*, 22 (8), 728-741 (1877).

4   Little, J. A Hitherto Undescribed Lesion as a Cause of Epistaxis. *Hospital Gazette*, 6, 5-6 (1879).

5   Kiesselbach, W. Über spontane Nasenblutungen. *Wiener klinische Wochenschrift*, 21, 375–377 (1884).

6   Jordanes. *The origin and deeds of the Goths*. Translated by Mierow, C. C. CreateSpace Independent Publishing Platform (2011).

MOUTH AND THROAT

BAD BREATH

If you are frequently offered mints, this chapter is for you.

Listerine mouthwash was originally spruiked as a floor cleaner, aftershave, deodorant and treatment for gonorrhoea. Quite bold claims for a mixture of a few essential oils dissolved in alcohol. Listerine might freshen your breath, but its dubious marketing track record leaves a very bad taste in the mouth.

The name Listerine is a nod to the British surgeon Joseph Lister (1827-1912), a pioneer of antiseptic surgery. In Lister's time, post-operative infections killed half of all patients undergoing major operations. Surgeons blamed infection on noxious vapours called miasma (from the Greek for 'pollution'). 'Infection prevention' meant opening the ward's windows to let in a fresh breeze.

But by the 1860s, revolution was afoot. French chemist Louis Pasteur was churning out extraordinary research that would ultimately lead to germ theory: the idea that infection with microorganisms like bacteria and viruses could cause disease. In 1865 while reading one of Pasteur's papers, Lister had a brainwave. Perhaps he could prevent infection by applying a substance to his patient's skin that would kill these newfangled germs? We now call these germ-killing substances antiseptics, from the Greek *anti septikos* ('against putrefaction'). Common antiseptics are high-concentration alcohols (such as in hand sanitising gel, or those wet swabs used to wipe your skin before an injection) and iodine (found in brown sore throat gargles and the fluid sloshed over your abdomen before a surgeon makes an incision, for example). Lister suspected that carbolic acid, a coal-tar derivative also known as phenol, might be an effective antiseptic based on an article he had read the year before:

> ... I was much struck with an account of the remarkable effects produced by carbolic acid upon the sewage of the town of Carlisle, the admixture of a very small portion not only preventing all odour from the lands irrigated with the refuse material, but [also] destroying the entozoa which usually infest cattle fed on such pastures.[1]

If carbolic acid could deodorise germ-ridden sewage and kill the intestinal worms in cows, maybe it could destroy microorganisms on human skin too?

Lister didn't have to wait long until he could test his theory. On August 12, 1865, an 11-year-old lad named James Greenlees was rushed to the Glasgow Royal Infirmary with a gruesome leg wound. A cart's wheel had rolled over his left leg, leaving a snapped shinbone poking through his skin. Lister successfully realigned the bone ends, but without amputation – the usual treatment for such a severe injury at that time – the open wound was sure to become infected. Since there was nothing to lose (except the boy's leg), Lister stuffed James's wound with surgical dressings soaked in carbolic acid. Four days later Lister gingerly plucked out the dressings. No infection. Thrilled, Lister packed in more carbolic acid-soaked dressings. After six weeks' treatment Greenlees' shinbone had knitted together without infection. Lister's findings, published in *The Lancet* in 1867, completely revolutionised surgical practice.[1] The use of antiseptics became routine in the operating theatre. Vats of carbolic acid were used to dowse surgeons' hands, instruments, operating tables and patients. Post-operative infection rates plummeted. Today Lister is widely regarded as the greatest surgical benefactor to mankind.

Across the Atlantic, Lister's work inspired Missouri-based chemist Joseph Lawrence to concoct his own antiseptic. By 1879, Lawrence had finalised the recipe for Listerine, his ethanol-based blend of essential oils extracted from thyme, eucalyptus, wintergreen and mint. Of note, it's the essential oils that give Listerine its antiseptic properties, not the ethanol. Alcohols need to be at least 60 per cent concentrated to have antiseptic properties. At only 25 per cent concentration, the ethanol in the concoction isn't strong enough to kill microorganisms; it's just used to dissolve the essential oils. Lawrence had greater ambitions for Listerine beyond the operating theatre. Keeping his formula secret, in 1881 Lawrence licensed *Listerine* to a local pharmacist, Jordan Lambert. It was initially marketed by the Lambert Pharmacal Company as a sort of wonder liquid, treating anything from dandruff to dysentery. But it wasn't until 1914 that a diluted version of Listerine became America's first over-the-counter mouthwash for bad breath.

Early sales were modest. Bad breath certainly existed but wasn't discussed in polite company. If Listerine was going to succeed as a mouthwash, consumers had to regard bad breath as a serious problem, even a disease. An obscure medical term already existed for bad breath: 'halitosis', from the Latin *halitus* (breath) and Greek *nosis* (disease). Physician Joseph William Howe had coined the term in his 1874 book *The breath and the diseases which give it fetid odor*, but the word hadn't really caught on. During a business meeting, Listerine's company chemist mentioned halitosis in passing to Gerald Lambert, Jordan Lambert's son who by this time was running the Lambert Pharmacal Company. In Gerard Lambert's words:

> When [the chemist] came into our room, I asked him if Listerine was good for bad breath. He excused himself for a moment and came back with a big book of newspaper clippings. He sat in a chair and I stood looking over his shoulder. He thumbed through the immense book. 'Here it is, Gerard. It says in this

clipping from the British *Lancet* that in cases of halitosis ...'
I interrupted, 'What is halitosis?' 'Oh,' he said, 'that is the
medical term for bad breath.' [The chemist] never knew what
had hit him. I bustled the poor old fellow out of the room.
'There,' I said, 'is something to hang our hat on.'[2]

Halitosis was exactly the euphemism Listerine needed to grow its
market. Bad breath was embarrassing to talk about, but halitosis
had a scholarly medical ring to it. This mouthwash was no longer
just a cosmetic breath-freshener, it was the pharmacological cure
for halitosis.

The company's advertising campaigns propelled halitosis
into the public consciousness. Halitosis was portrayed as an
undiagnosed epidemic, the unspoken obstacle thwarting your
dreams of success, wealth and love. Listerine's advertisements
were shameless: 'Are you unpopular with your own children?';
'They talk about you behind your back'; 'Let the tide take her
out ... I won't!' (said by a man on the beach watching his female
companion paddling in the ocean); and the most direct of all:
'Halitosis makes you unpopular'.

In 1923 Listerine launched its infamous 'Often a bridesmaid
but never a bride' campaign. Advertisements featured a forlorn
woman dubbed Edna or Eleanor who was unaware that her
halitosis was preventing her from finding true love. *Listerine* took
out full-page adverts featuring a weeping bridesmaid accompanied
by the caption:

Edna's case was really a pathetic one. Like every woman, her
primary ambition was to marry. Most of the girls of her set
were married – or about to be. Yet not one possessed more
grace or charm or loveliness than she.

And as her birthdays crept gradually toward that tragic
thirty-mark, marriage seemed farther from her life than ever.

She was often a bridesmaid but never a bride.

> That's the insidious thing about halitosis (unpleasant
> breath). You, yourself, rarely know when you have it. And even
> your closest friends won't tell you.

As a consequence of encouraging halitophobia (yes, this is a medical term), *Listerine's* US revenue skyrocketed from $115,000 in 1922 to over $8 million by 1929.[3]

Attempting to replicate *Listerine's* success, some companies tried to medicalise problems that their products could ostensibly cure (for example, *bromodosis* [smelly feet], or *homotosis* [bad taste in home furnishing]). Other companies blatantly invented maladies to shift their products (like 'office hips', 'vacation knees', or 'spoon-food face').[4] Fear-based medical advertising intensified in the 1930s: 'Can bad toilet paper lead to surgery?' (Scott Paper Company 1931); 'Will the jaw atrophy unless exercised with chewing gum?' (Dentyne, 1934); 'Might poor quality bandages lead to amputation?' (Johnson & Johnson, 1936).[5]

Crackdowns on brazen advertising claims saw these egregious campaigns gradually diminish. Today, Listerine is sold as just a mouthwash that: 'Kills germs that cause bad breath'. Don't use it as a hair tonic, don't clean your floors with it, and certainly don't bathe your gonorrhoea-infected genitals in it.

*

Contrary to the wisdom of 19th century dental journals, bad breath does not result from 'want of exercise, too much worry and mental strain' or 'too much sensuality'.[6] What *will* cause bad breath, however, is oral bacteria.

The human mouth is riddled with bacteria. Tongue grooves provide sheltered cul-de-sacs for bacterial colonies to settle. Tight spaces between your 32 teeth offer further snug accommodation. Bacteria thrive on food remnants wedged between your teeth and sitting on the back of your tongue, marinating in saliva.

Like all living creatures, bacteria need to produce energy to survive. Humans' energy-making reactions rely on oxygen, which is why we breathe. Other so-called anaerobic organisms, like the bacteria that cause bad breath, make energy via chemical reactions that don't use oxygen. Fermentation is one such anaerobic reaction. We can thank fermentation for giving us beer, bread, cheese and wine. But fermentation isn't always pleasant. Gas gangrene is the result of a wound infection by anaerobic bacteria, usually *Clostridium perfringens*. Under your skin, these bacteria produce tiny bubbles as they ferment your tissue, similar to the bubbles that form during beer fermentation. Touching a wound with gas gangrene is a memorable experience: the trapped pockets of gas make the flesh feel like bubble wrap. Less deadly but similarly unpleasant is Sweden's infamous fermented fish 'delicacy' *surströmming* (from *sur* 'sour' and *strömming* 'Baltic herring'), crowned the most putrid smelling food on earth by a 2002 Japanese study.[7] Food critic Wolfgang Fassbender asserted that 'The biggest challenge when eating *surströmming* is to vomit after the first bite, and not before.' And to finish our foul fermentation list: bad breath.

During fermentation oral bacteria release putrid products called volatile organic compounds. 'Volatile' describes the compounds' readiness to evaporate at normal room temperature and waft as gases from your mouth. One such gas is hydrogen sulfide, present in sewers and swamp gas, which smells like rotten eggs. Another is methyl mercaptan, which is also present in flatulence and produced as a by-product of asparagus digestion (your kidneys remove the methyl mercaptan from your blood via urine, giving it the unmistakable 'asparagus pee' odour). Dimethyl sulfide is another particularly malodorous volatile organic compound which smells like a rotting animal carcass. The plant 'dead horse arum lily', *Helicodiceros muscivorus*, releases dimethyl sulfide to attract flies which it relies on for pollination.

It's normal to have some anaerobic bacteria fermenting away in your mouth. An overgrowth of them, however, makes your breath smell like a can of *surströmming*.

Constantly making and swallowing saliva is key to controlling your mouth's anaerobic bacterial population. Waves of saliva dislodge bacteria which you then remove by swallowing. You produce half to one litre (one to two pints) of saliva every day. Sitting still reading this book your saliva will be dripping out at about 0.4 millilitres per minute. Chewing or eating something will increase saliva secretion tenfold, but during sleep, the rate drops to 0.1 millilitre per minute. Plus, as pillow drool proves, you stop swallowing. Overnight your oral bacteria enjoy an unfettered fermentation fiesta. The 'morning breath' emanating from your yawning mouth is due to the mass release of accumulated volatile organic compounds.

Anything that dries up your saliva will allow bacterial populations to boom. That means more fermentation, more volatile organic compounds and worse breath. Certain medications, like diuretics and anti-nausea drugs, decrease saliva production as a side-effect. Going for long periods without food stops eating-associated saliva surges. Despite its bad smell, 'fasting breath' may save your life. In 2006, researchers explored a novel technique for detecting trapped people after earthquakes: their bad breath.[8] They reasoned that after hours entombed in rubble without eating, the victims' dry mouths would be releasing industrial quantities of volatile organic compounds. A handheld device called a gas chromatograph could detect these compounds when waved over the ruins of a crumbled building. To determine what gases the chromatograph should be seeking, the researchers needed a sample population of fasting people's breath. Seven monks on Greece's Mount Athos volunteered. After 63 hours without food, each monk's breath was analysed. The most specific fasting human breath compound was acetone, present in the monks' breath at 30 times the concentration of well-fed controls. Acetone is the same chemical that gives nail polish remover its characteristic smell. Acetone also dissolves superglue. Emergency departments always keep some on hand to unstick the fingers of hapless DIY-ers.

People with 'poor oral hygiene' (the euphemistic term doctors use to describe patients with rotten teeth) are more likely to have bad breath. Unbrushed teeth quickly develop a film of bacteria and food called plaque. The bacteria that enjoy living in plaque also enjoy making acids. Acid fizzles away the underlying tooth to form cavities, which trap food and provide further refuges for bacterial colonies. More bacteria, worse breath.

Bacteria don't have to be in your mouth to cause bad breath. Infected tonsils or sinuses brimming with pus are obvious reservoirs of odour-producing bacteria. Particularly among adventurous children, infected foreign bodies trapped up the nose can release foul odours from the nostrils. A festering lung abscess can seep its unpleasant odours into your airways, released each time you exhale.

Characteristic breath aromas can be used to diagnose diseases. When you breathe, your lungs release gaseous waste chemicals from your blood, mainly carbon dioxide. Some diseases cause specific chemicals to accumulate in your blood. If these chemicals are volatile like carbon dioxide, they'll be released via your lungs in your breath. One such example is ammonia, which accumulates in kidney failure. The resulting 'ammonia breath' smells like urine and tastes strongly metallic. If you suddenly smell freshly mown hay while roaming a hospital, there's probably a patient with liver failure nearby. A damaged liver can't filter certain sweet musty-smelling volatile chemicals from the blood. Measurement of other exhaled gases can be used to make diagnoses like alcohol intoxication (blowing into a breathalyser) and fructose or lactose malabsorption (hydrogen breath tests).

What about that acetone in the Mount Athos monks' breath? When the body runs out of glucose to provide fuel, it starts breaking down fats in a process called ketosis. Acetone is one of the products of ketosis. As a volatile compound, acetone leaves your body via your breath, giving it that nail polish remover smell. Besides prolonged fasting, acetone breath from ketosis can result from very low carbohydrate diets, or occur in people with diabetes who don't take enough insulin.

Eating pungent foods will result in equally pungent breath. Coffee has a double-whammy bad breath effect: a powerful odour plus a diuretic effect which dries out your mouth. Members of the onion family like garlic and leek contain smelly sulfur-containing volatile compounds that coat your mouth and immediately waft from it. But you don't even have to chew garlic to get garlic breath; swallowing a clove whole would still result in halitosis. Garlic's sulfur compounds are released into your bloodstream after being digested. Since they're volatile, for the next 24 hours the stinky compounds seep from your blood into your lungs and escape via your breath. They also become incorporated into your sweat and emanate from your armpits. No amount of tooth brushing will cure garlic breath: it's the result of internal chemical reactions, not a wayward chunk of garlic between your back teeth. Oils in spices like cumin have the same effect.

If you avoid whiffy foods and control your oral bacteria, you should be able to maintain fresh breath. Starve the bacteria by flossing away trapped food, physically dislodge them by brushing, and consider annihilating them with an antiseptic mouthwash. What's less straightforward, due to social niceties, is discovering that you've got bad breath in the first place. Dentist Dr John Codman lyrically outlined this dilemma in his 1879 essay 'Foul Breath' published in the *American Journal of Dental Science*:

> Oftentimes we meet the intelligent and the able, the profound and the artistic. They may have earnest and noble faces; their conversation be rapt and energetic; but we turn away in disgust from the foul odour that comes in the same breath with words of affection, of wisdom and love … Verily, have I not been offended beyond measure, in dental meetings and among dentists, by dentists themselves?[6]

A reader's reply to Dr Codman's essay, published in the subsequent issue of the journal, offered this sage advice:

> A candid mentor is most useful in such cases. It is not in good taste to consult one's acquaintance on the subject. An evasive answer is almost invariably given; and then too the sufferer from this malady is, as a rule, unaware of its existence. Consult your wife, sister, mother, and do this frequently, not waiting for them to call your attention to the trouble but invite criticism. The olfactories of women are more sensitive than those of men.[9]

SUMMARY: Healthy mouths contain anaerobic bacteria. Populations can boom when your mouth dries out. The stinky volatile products of their cumulative fermentation cause bad breath.

AND ALSO ...

Handing it to Ignaz Semmelweis

Before we came to understand germ theory – the idea that microorganisms like bacteria cause disease – surgeons were famously filthy. Why wash your surgical gown? Are not the accumulated blood stains testament to your surgical experience? The sickly odour pervading grimy operating theatres was lovingly referred to as the 'good old surgical stink'. Pus was considered a normal part of wound healing. One unwashed probe would be used to examine the suppurating wounds of all patients on a ward round.

Early advocates for improved sanitation were mocked and dismissed. Consider the tale of Hungarian physician Ignaz Semmelweis, who was appointed to the Vienna General Hospital in 1846. The hospital had two maternity clinics where healthcare staff were trained. Medical students were taught in the first clinic, midwifery students in the second. Pregnant women were allocated to each clinic on alternate days. The two clinics were identical, with one major exception: the mortality rate. Between 1840 to 1846, an average of 10 per cent of women in the first clinic, the one where the medical students trained, died. Women in the second clinic, under the trainee midwives' care, only had a four per cent mortality rate. In both clinics, most women were dying from puerperal fever: a disease that we now know to be caused by bacterial infection of the reproductive tract.

Nobody could explain the excess deaths from puerperal fever in the first clinic – until Semmelweis entered the fray. Semmelweis noticed a key difference in the medical and midwifery students' timetables. The medical students started each day by performing autopsies of women who had recently died from puerperal fever. Then, without washing their hands, they proceeded directly to the first clinic to perform a vaginal examination on each patient, as required by their training program. Conversely, midwifery students were not required to perform autopsies or routine vaginal examinations.

Semmelweis proposed that the transmission of 'morbid matter' on the medical students' hands was to blame for the first clinic's higher mortality rate. Don't mock him for calling it 'morbid matter': it would be another 20 years before Pasteur's work would reveal the role of microorganisms in causing disease. Semmelweis was right, but for the wrong reasons. Besides a quick rub on their surgical gown, a medical student's hands went directly from a dead woman's festering womb to the vaginas of every woman in their clinic.

Acting on this morbid matter idea, in May 1847 Semmelweis introduced a policy requiring medical students to wash their hands with chlorinated lime (essentially a bleach solution) on entering the first clinic. Semmelweis had no idea that chlorinated lime had antiseptic properties; he selected it because it most effectively removed the smell (which presumably carried the morbid matter, he reasoned) of rotting corpses from the students' skin. The result was remarkable. The first clinic's mortality rate plummeted from a peak of 18.27 per cent in April 1847 to just 1.2 per cent in July.[10]

Despite the success of Semmelweis's intervention, his ideas about the importance of cleanliness met firm opposition. Disease was still thought to be caused by an imbalance of bodily fluids called humours, not physically transmissible morbid matter. Outraged surgeons took umbrage to the inference that they were 'unclean' or were somehow to blame for causing disease in their patients. Disbelieved and derided, Semmelweis's mental health deteriorated and in 1865 he was involuntarily committed to a psychiatric hospital. He died a fortnight later, aged just 47, from a gangrenous hand wound.

Get a whiff of this, predators

Tobacco hornworms aren't worms and don't have horns. They do, however, eat tobacco leaves which are packed with the poisonous bitter alkaloid nicotine (see *Taste and smell (loss of)*, page 134). Nicotine is a natural pesticide. It's so toxic that very few creatures can survive eating tobacco leaves. You'd feel queasy after eating just a few tobacco leaves. Children have died from poisoning after ingesting just 60 milligrams of nicotine (the equivalent of six cigarettes). Tobacco hornworms, however, with a nicotine tolerance 750 times greater than humans, can chow through a leafy tobacco lunch without issue. Unlike humans, hornworms don't seek out nicotine to get a buzz (in fact digesting the nicotine is energy-consuming and makes the worms drowsy). Instead, their tobacco leaf diet is a defence mechanism. Scientists have discovered a gene that allows the tobacco hornworm to puff digested nicotine from its pores 'like toxic halitosis', as researcher Ian Baldwin put it.[11] Predators like wolf spiders are deterred by the nicotine breath and seek their dinner elsewhere.

ENDNOTES

1   Lister, J. On a New Method of Treating Compound Fracture, Abscess, &c., with Observations on the Conditions of Suppuration. *The Lancet*, 336–339 (1867).

2   Lambert, G. B. *All Out of Step: A Personal Chronicle*. Doubleday (1956).

3   Twitchel, J. B. *20 Ads that Shook the World: The Century's Most Groundbreaking Advertising and how it changed us*. All Crown Publishers, p. 64 (2000).

4   Ewen, S. *Captains of Consciousness. Advertising and the Social Roots of the Consumer Culture*. McGraw Hill (1976).

5   Goodrum, C. & Dalrymple, H. *Advertising in America, The first two hundred years*. Harry N. Abrams (1990).

6   Codman, J. T. Foul breath. *American Journal of Dental Science*, 12 (12), 529-542 (1879).

7   Koizumi, T. Hakkou Ha Chikara Nari. *NHK Kouza* (2002).

8   Statheropoulos, M. et al. Analysis of expired air of fasting male monks at Mount Athos. *Journal of Chromatography B*, 832 (2), 274–279 (2006).

9   Remarks on Article on Foul Breath. *American Journal of Dental Science*, 13 (1), 45-46 (1879).

10 Shorter, E. Ignaz Semmelweis: The etiology, concept, and prophylaxis of childbed fever. *Medical History*, 28 (3), 334 (1984).

11 Kumar, P. et al. Natural history-driven, plant-mediated RNAi-based study reveals CYP6B46's role in a nicotine-mediated antipredator herbivore defense. *Proceedings of the National Academy of Sciences*, 111 (4), 1245–1252 (2013).

TASTE AND SMELL (LOSS OF)
Mud cake may as well be mud when you've got a head cold.

John Harvey Kellogg, doctor and cereal creator, deliberately invented corn flakes to be tasteless and underwhelming. 'The diet should be made abstemious,' he stressed in his 1887 book *Plain Facts for Old and Young*: 'Eat fruits, grains, milk and vegetables ... they are wholesome and unstimulating.'[1] Kellogg shunned flavoursome foods for a rather unusual reason: he believed that they caused sexual arousal.

> A man that lives on pork, fine-flour bread, rich pies and cakes,
> and condiments, drinks tea and coffee, and uses tobacco,
> might as well try to fly as to be chaste in thought.

As a devout Seventh Day Adventist, Kellogg abhorred 'sexual excesses', a term which covered everything besides intercourse for the purposes of procreation. 'Nothing tends so powerfully to keep passions in abeyance as a simple diet, free from condiments.' Kellogg claimed that certain incriminating taste preferences were characteristic of a sexual transgressor. Masturbation, a habit he considered to be 'the most dangerous of all sexual abuses', should be suspected in those with a 'disgust for simple food', a predilection for 'eating slate-pencils', or an 'extreme fondness for unnatural, hurtful, and irritating foods':

> Nearly all [people who masturbate] are greatly attached to salt, pepper, spices, cinnamon, cloves, vinegar, mustard, horse-radish, and similar articles, and use them in most inordinate quantities. A boy or girl who is constantly eating cloves or cinnamon, or who will eat salt in quantities without other food, gives good occasion for suspicion.

In 1876 Kellogg was appointed medical director at the Battle Creek Sanitarium in Michigan, a hospital-cum-health spa run according to strict Adventist values. Kellogg preached and prescribed an unstimulating vegetarian diet to all his patients, including rock-hard hunks of bread. After a woman cracked her dentures trying to gnaw through the rusk and threatened to sue, Kellogg 'began to think that we ought to have a ready-cooked food which would not break people's teeth'.[2] Corn flakes resulted from his experiments with toasting and shaving various grains. Kellogg's original corn flakes were even blander than the modern version (if that were possible). No sugar, no salt: just toasted scales of corn. Despite tasting like cardboard, the flakes were an instant hit among his patients. Kellogg's brother Will, the sanitarium's bookkeeper, smelt a business opportunity in commercialising the flakes. Will suggested tweaking the recipe with a sprinkle of sugar to broaden their appeal. You can imagine his brother's response. After a bitter legal battle, Will went solo and began mass-marketing sugared corn flakes to the US in 1906.

John Kellogg died in 1943, a decade before Kellogg's released Sugar Smacks: toasted puffs of sweetened wheat promoted by a menacing clown. No food could be further from John Kellogg's frugal dietary principles. For every 100 grams (3.5 ounces) of Sugar Smacks cereal, 55 grams (2 ounces) were sugar. As for the name, the 'sugar' was for obvious reasons, the 'smacks' presumably because the sweetness was as subtle as a slap in the face. When sugar fell out of fashion in the 1980s, clever marketers tried to boost the cereal's health rating with a sly renaming: Honey Smacks. The recipe was identical, but since honey is considered 'natural', the rechristening gave the product a veneer of health. Although Kellogg's marketing was tasteless, its sickly-sweet cereal certainly was not.

*

Your sense of taste contributes relatively little to a food's flavour. Here's an experiment to prove it. Grab a bag of jelly beans and a peg. With nose pegged and eyes shut, fish out a random jellybean from the bag and start chewing. All you'll taste is sweetness: you won't be able to identify if you're chewing a strawberry or orange jellybean, for example. Unplug your nose and suddenly the fruity flavour will become apparent. Now, open your mouth and your eyes and use a mirror to look at the colour of the bean mush on your tongue. Having identified the pink colour, for example, you might notice that the berry flavour becomes more intense as you finish chewing and swallow.

Flavour is a combination of a food's smell, taste, colour, temperature, texture (or 'mouth feel' as it's often unappealingly termed) and other intangible qualities like your environment and mood. A ripe banana plucked and eaten straight from a tree will have a far superior flavour to the banana you wolf down at your desk before an afternoon of back-to-back meetings.

The jellybean experiment proves that smell, much more than taste, gives food its flavour. When you complain that you've lost your sense of taste, what you've actually lost is your sense of smell.

Your nasal cavities reach all the way up to between your eyebrows. Here, a thin perforated bone called the cribriform plate (Latin for 'sieve-like') is the only thing separating inhaled air from your brain. The tiny holes in the bone allow scent-detecting nerves to protrude like weeds from your brain into your nose. The nerve endings form a patch about the size of a postage stamp on the roof of your nasal cavities. Odour molecules released by things around you, like pine trees or wet dogs, bind to the nerve endings as they waft to the roof of your nose. Different nerve endings can detect different odour molecules. Your brain interprets the patterns of nerve activation as the smell of Christmas tree or damp dachshund, for example. The human nose is capable of detecting over one trillion different smells.

Temporary or permanent loss of smell can severely affect your enjoyment of food. As you chew, odour molecules emanate from the food in your mouth and ascend via the back of your throat to stimulate your nose's scent receptors. If your nose is stuffed with globs of mucous, those receptors are equally stuffed: the thick slime physically prevents odour molecules from reaching the nerve endings. As the mucous dries up, your sense of smell returns.

Anosmia is the medical term for an inability to smell. Some people are born anosmic, like the poet William Wordsworth (he was being entirely metaphorical when he said 'the flower that smells the sweetest is shy and lowly'). Other people are rendered anosmic by head trauma. A hefty whack to the head can shear off the scent-detecting nerves passing through the bony holes in your cribriform plate. Anosmia can also be the first sign of Parkinson's disease, appearing years before any tremor manifests. The nerve damage seen in Parkinson's disease begins in the part of the brain just above the cribriform plate.

*

Your tongue can detect five primary tastes: sour, salty, sweet, bitter, and umami (savoury taste). Combinations of these tastes contribute to a food's unique taste profile. Your high school biology textbook may have contained a 'tongue map': a diagram depicting a tongue divided into segments according to what taste is detected there. Alas, tongue maps are as scientifically valid as horoscopes. Daub some jam or peanut butter on various parts of your tongue and this falsehood will become immediately evident – you can detect all five primary tastes anywhere on your tongue.

Go to the mirror and poke out your tongue. See the taste buds? The answer is a definite no, unless you're looking at your tongue's reflection through a high-powered microscope. Those pink bumps you can see are called papillae, from the Latin word for nipple. The easiest papillae to visualise are the circumvallate papillae: those 10 to 14 chunky bumps arranged in a V-shape right at the back of your tongue. Mushroom-shaped fungiform papillae occupy the front of your tongue. Wiggle your tongue to one side and note the vertical ridges made by leaf-shaped foliate papillae. Your tongue's 10,000 or so taste buds, not visible to the naked eye, line the sides of all of these papillae. Further taste buds line your cheeks, the roof of your mouth and the top of your oesophagus.

Taste buds regenerate about every 10 days. So, if you burn your tongue on a melted cheese sandwich, those damaged buds should be able to fully appreciate another (adequately cooled, this time) in about a week and a half.

Taste buds serve an important survival function: they encourage animals to seek tasty nutrient-rich food and avoid potential poisons. Taste bud quotas differ among animal species depending on their diets. Carnivores have fewer than 500 taste buds, most of which are tuned to detect bitterness to discourage dining on rancid meat. Meat-eaters are also oblivious to sweet tastes. Sugars don't form part of a lion's natural diet, hence having sweet-sensitive taste buds would be pointless. Herbivores lie at the other end of the spectrum with about 25,000 taste buds. Plant-eaters need a finely tuned sense of taste to detect traces of toxins in the tons of greenery they endlessly chow down on every day. When an elephant shoves an entire limb of an acacia tree into its mouth, its superior sense of taste allows it to detect a bitter single toxic leaf hidden among the foliage. Fish are particularly well-endowed with taste buds.

Fish not only have taste buds in their mouth but also lining the sides of their body to sample chemicals in the water. Catfish have 175,000 taste buds: the most of any animal. Prowling murky water with zero visibility means that they rely on their sense of taste to hunt down food.

Taste buds are shaped like garlic bulbs. Each taste bud contains 50 to 150 taste cells arranged like cloves. The taste bud is topped with a tuft of hair-like projections that waft about in the saliva coating your tongue. When you chew a mouthful of food, your churning jaw action mixes the food in your saliva and distributes it across your tongue. Your taste buds' hairs detect the chemicals in that gloopy soup and set off reactions in the taste cells beneath. Importantly, the hairs can only detect a chemical when they're bathed in it. If you sprinkled sugar, salt and bleach powder on a dry tongue, they would be equally as tasteless as gravel. A network of nerves extends like roots from the base of each taste bud. These nerves convey your taste buds' chemical activity to your brain, which interprets the data as taste.

How do your taste buds 'know' if a food is sweet or salty? Well, consider how any of our other special senses 'know' what they have detected. Your eyes can identify colour based on detecting wavelengths of light, while your ears rely on sound wave frequencies to detect a sound's pitch. Instead of light wavelengths or air vibrations, your taste buds detect tastes based on a food's chemical properties. Specific chemicals are associated with each of the five primary tastes. The different chemicals trigger different chemical reactions in your taste buds, allowing them to 'know' what they're tasting.

Sour tastes are due to acids. Put anything with a low pH on your tongue – vinegar, kiwi fruit, Greek yoghurt, your stomach contents (see *Nausea and vomiting*, page 177) – and your brain will tell you it's sour. It's the hydrogen ion in particular that sets off the sour-signalling chemical reaction in your taste buds. A surge of saliva invariably floods your mouth after taking a bite of something sour. Your body releases the extra drool (which is more than 99 per cent water) to dilute the acid in your sour snack to protect your teeth from acid erosion. Imagine crunching some salt and vinegar chips. Is saliva pooling in your mouth? If not, imagine quartering a lemon and taking a bite of its juicy yellow flesh. Merely imagining eating a sour food is usually enough to get your salivary glands pumping. This is a conditioned response from previous encounters with sour foods. If your brain thinks you're about to hoe into some citrus, it preemptively squirts out some protective saliva.

Casu marzu is a Sardinian cheese prized for its tangy, sour taste. The sheep's milk cheese gets its unique flavour from the live maggots that infest it. As the fly larvae munch on the cheese, acids in their digestive tract break down the cheese fats. The maggot excrement gives casu marzu (literally 'putrid cheese') its acidic taste. Sardinians traditionally eat the cheese with the larvae still alive and wriggling. More squeamish diners pick out the maggots. Others suggest sealing the cheese in a paper bag to asphyxiate the maggots. At first, the suffocating larvae will spring from the cheese, making a popping sound as they collide with the bag. When the popping stops, signifying successful maggot extermination, you can remove the cheese and enjoy it (I use the term 'enjoy' very loosely) spread on flatbread, maggot corpses included. Not surprisingly, the cheese, inexplicably considered to be an aphrodisiac and often served at weddings, has been banned by the European Union. Permitting flies to frolic in cheese can riddle it with disease-causing bacteria. Plus, if the maggots survive the acidic pool of your stomach, they can cause abdominal pain, nausea and vomiting as they burrow into the walls of your intestines.

What do anchovies, olives, and Vegemite have in common? The letter V, a black colour, and a hefty salt content. Salty tastes are due to dissolved metal ions, also known as electrolytes. Sodium chloride (table salt) is the most common electrolyte we eat. We don't even bother specifying the elements of sodium and chloride: we just call it salt. It's specifically the sodium ions that taste salty. But other metal ions besides sodium taste salty too. Potassium ions, in the form of potassium chloride powder, can be sprinkled on fries as a salt substitute for people who need to limit their sodium intake for health reasons, like high blood pressure. Patients prescribed tablets containing the mood-stabilising metal lithium often complain of its salty taste and feeling perpetually thirsty.

Salt's moreish taste motivates animals to seek the ions they require to maintain their body's electrolyte balance. Deer and giraffes flock to natural salt sources to lick up their electrolyte quotas. Ibexes have been spotted in Northern Italy scaling near-vertical dam walls to suck up the rock's salty goodness. Pregnancy can cause fluctuations in a woman's electrolyte levels, resulting in seemingly random cravings for popcorn and pretzels. Unlike ibexes, humans no longer need to scavenge for salt thanks to its surfeit in our modern processed diets. Your body only needs a teaspoon of salt per day (about six grams, which contains two grams of sodium) but most people easily ingest double that. Salt is appealing even when you're not deficient, an evolutionary hangover that explains why it's so difficult to stop at just one potato chip.

Sweet tastes are produced by several chemicals, most notably sugars. Sugars are carbohydrates which, as the name suggests, are molecules containing carbon hydrated by water (which is hydrogen and oxygen). Sucrose is the sugar you stir into your coffee. Fruits and honey are sweet thanks to the sugar fructose, while lactose is the sugar which gives milk its sweetness. Sugar molecules are energy-dense.

Evolutionarily speaking, our sweet tooth encouraged efficient foraging for high calorie fruits rather than wasting our efforts preparing boiled bark. Many plants evolved to bear sweet fruits or flowers filled with sugary nectar to tempt creatures to eat them, thereby helping the plant to reproduce. When a bee sucks up a flower's nectar it becomes dusted with pollen. If a bird eats a berry, it will later expel the seeds in its guano. By exploiting another creature's sweet tooth to spread its pollen and seeds, a plant's germination range can extend significantly.

Not all sweet-tasting chemicals are sugars. Sugar substitutes like saccharin, aspartame and sorbitol are non-carbohydrate chemicals that happen to taste sweet. Several convicted murderers have admitted to spiking their victim's beverage with a less conventional sugar substitute: ethylene glycol, more commonly known as antifreeze. Unlike most poisons, which tend to taste bitter, the syrupy sweet antifreeze is easy to mix into coffee and cocktails undetected. The antidote to antifreeze poisoning is a second tasty beverage: alcohol. In the hospital setting we give pharmaceutical grade ethanol through a drip, but drinking gin, vodka, whisky or any other strong spirit will do the job nicely. Alcohol acts as a decoy: your liver preferentially breaks down the booze rather than the antifreeze. Ethylene glycol itself isn't lethal: it's the chemicals produced as your liver breaks it down that will kill you. Preoccupying your liver with breaking down alcohol will buy your kidneys enough time to harmlessly remove the ethylene glycol from your system via your urine.

Chloroform is another lethally sweet chemical that tastes 40 times sweeter than sugar. Don't test this out: just 10 millilitres can cause death via respiratory failure or cardiac arrest. At lower doses, chloroform causes unconsciousness. Chloroform-soaked rags held to a patient's nose were used in the Victorian age as an anaesthetic. It takes a few minutes of deep inhalation before you pass out; the Hollywood version of immediate collapse after touching the damp cloth to the target's face is a tad exaggerated.

Bitter foods are generally derived from plants. Many forms of flora evolved to incorporate acrid chemicals into their foliage and fruit to dissuade animals from eating them. This strategy fails miserably when it comes to the highly sought-after bitter alkaloids found in coffee beans (caffeine), cinchona bark (quinine, used in tonic water) and cocoa beans (theobromine). More successful employment of the 'don't eat me I'm bitter' strategy is observed among those plants whose bitter alkaloids will make you drop dead if ingested, like the strychnine tree, hemlock, deadly nightshade, monkshood and tobacco (see *Bad breath*, page 124). Potassium cyanide is an exceedingly toxic chemical found in plants including cassava and lima beans. Its bitter-almond smell is well-documented, but because ingestion causes death within minutes, nobody has ever survived to document its taste. The mystery was solved in 2006 when an Indian goldsmith known only as M. P. Prasad hastily scrawled a suicide note after eating it: 'Doctors, potassium cyanide. I have tasted it. It burns the tongue and tastes acrid.'[3] Somewhere between delicious (coffee) and deadly (cyanide) lie the compounds that impart bitterness to various fruits and vegetables, like cucurbitacin (gourds and cucumbers), humulone (hops) and glucosinolates (members of the Brassicaceae family, which includes broccoli, cabbage and horseradish). Flavonoids like naringin (found in grapefruit) and anthocyanins (think red and blue fruits and vegetables, like rhubarb, grapes and cranberries) carry a bitter bite too.

Bitter foods tend to be more popular among grandparents than grandchildren. Taste buds deteriorate and become less sensitive with age. Foods that were unbearably bitter to you as a child may taste increasingly palatable as you mature. Rather than juvenile stubbornness, children's dislike of all things green may have evolved as a protective trait. Plants – poisonous or otherwise – tend to taste somewhat bitter. Until you hone your botanical identification skills, it's smart to avoid eating all plants to circumvent sudden death-by-salad. Taste buds that are super-sensitive to bitter deter children from experimenting with potentially lethal plants. Later, when your taste buds settle down to adult detection parameters, the mild bitterness of broccoli and beer becomes enjoyable.

If you don't trust your own taste buds to detect poisons, why not employ a human guinea pig to do it for you? Throughout history, powerful people with poisoning paranoia have done just that. Roman emperor Claudius required his eunuch servant Halotus to trot along to every banquet as his official taste tester. The plan backfired: Halotus was implicated in Claudius's murder by poisoned mushroom in 54 AD. Adolf Hitler forced 15 young girls to sample his food for poison during the final years of World War II. Margot Wolk was the only food taster who survived the war; Soviet soldiers killed the other 14 girls. In 2014, at the age of 95, Wolk described the terrifying ordeal in an interview with German TV station RBB:

> We had to eat it all up ... then we had to wait an hour, and every time we were frightened that we were going to be ill. We used to cry like dogs because we were so glad to have survived.[4]

Umami is roughly translated from Japanese as 'deliciousness'. If you've ever enjoyed the savoury taste of aged Parmesan, gravy or caramelised meat, you'd no doubt vouch for the translation's accuracy. Umami's addictiveness might explain why cheese is the most shoplifted food in the world: when an umami craving strikes, it's tough to resist. Umami was the most recent primary taste to be identified. In 1908, a chemist at Tokyo University named Kikunae Ikeda was trying to isolate the chemical responsible for the meaty taste of dashi, a staple stock in Japanese cuisine infused with kombu (kelp). Repeated experiments treating and evaporating the seaweed eventually yielded tiny crystals. When Ikeda took a taste, his mouth filled with the distinctive savoury taste he'd been seeking.

Molecular analysis revealed Ikeda's wonder chemical to be an amino acid called glutamate. Amino acids are the building blocks of proteins, hence umami being ubiquitous among high-protein food like meat and cheese. Slow cooking or fermenting a food can release extra glutamate to enhance a food's umami taste. In 1909, Ikeda mass-produced a condiment called ajinomoto (meaning 'essence of taste'). It was basically powdered umami: glutamate with sodium, also known as monosodium glutamate or MSG. The magic meaty powder gained traction throughout Asia, particularly as an additive in Chinese cooking. In the West, MSG was demonised in the 1960s as the cause of 'Chinese restaurant syndrome': an alleged symptom cluster of headache, sweating and skin-flushing following an MSG-laden Chinese meal. The syndrome has as much science behind it as the tongue map. Double-blinded studies have failed to demonstrate any link between MSG and adverse symptoms.[5]

*

To put all the taste science together, imagine sitting down to a meal at a fast food joint. You begin with a fistful of salted fries. As the sodium ions dissolve into your saliva, their salty taste encourages you to take a sip of lemonade. Sucrose molecules flood your taste buds, triggering a pleasant sweet sensation. The low pH of citric acid in the lemonade leaves a refreshing sour aftertaste. As you take a bite of a cheesy, meaty hamburger, your mouth fills with the delectable umami taste of glutamate. But suddenly a sharp bitter tang makes you spit out the bite in disgust. Peering into your burger you spy a half-eaten slice of cucurbitacin-packed pickle hiding beneath the beef patty. At times like this, John Harvey Kellogg's advice to stick to a simple diet, free from condiments, seems like a good idea.

SUMMARY: Your taste buds can detect five primary tastes: sour, salty, sweet, bitter, and umami. Each taste is associated with a class of chemicals that trigger specific reactions in your tastebuds. You perceive these reactions as taste.

AND ALSO …

What about spice?

Spiciness isn't a taste: it's a sensation of pain. Your taste buds don't recognise chemicals like capsaicin that make food spicy. Instead, the chemicals in chillies set off pain receptors in your mouth. Technically, it's impossible for anything to 'taste' spicy, though when fluid is pouring from every pore and facial orifice after accidentally nibbling a ghost pepper, this nuance hardly matters.

Astronauts in orbit suffer from chronic nasal congestion. Without gravity, mucous that would usually drain from their nose and sinuses pools in their head. Their stuffy noses render most food tasteless unless it's exceptionally heavily seasoned. Salt and pepper are available, but only in liquid form lest the grains float free and jam the craft's equipment. Spicy shrimp cocktail – freeze-dried prawns with powdered horseradish sauce – is routinely cited by astronauts as the most delicious food on the NASA menu. While piloting the *Endeavour* in 1995, astronaut Bill Gregory ate a shrimp cocktail with each of his 48 meals onboard. Gregory based his repetitive menu on the precedent set by six-time shuttle veteran Story Musgrave who ate shrimp cocktails three times a day whenever he was in orbit. Musgrave knew that once an astronaut had tasted the shrimp cocktail, they'd want to eat nothing else. Shrimp cocktails were so coveted in orbit that Musgrave advised his colleagues to copy his three-meals-a-day order so they didn't steal his. The prawns, coated with horseradish's bitter glucosinolates and spicy, pain-inducing compounds, offered a flavour experience that was out of this world.

Tasting the air

Snakes, lizards, and many mammals have a specialised chemical detector in their nose called Jacobson's organ. They use it to detect aerosolised pheromones squirted out by prey, predators and potential mates. Snakes protrude their tongue to sample the air before dabbing it upon their Jacobson's organ to 'taste' it. Horses jut their neck forward and curl back their upper lip to expose their Jacobson's organ. Humans can't detect pheromones because we don't possess a functional Jacobson's organ (except for people called Jacobson, in whom technically every organ is 'Jacobson's organ').

How sweet is too sweet?

In 1996, scientists at the University of Lyon, in central France, developed an artificial sweetener estimated to be up to 300,000 times sweeter than table sugar. They called it lugduname, from the Latin for 'Lyon'. Hypothetically, if you had a 27-gram (0.95-ounce) serving of Honey Smacks as the box suggests, 15 grams (0.5 ounces) of that would be sugar. Replace the sugar with lugduname and you'd only need 0.00005 grams of the sweetener for the same level of sweetness. Alternatively, if you replaced the sugar with the same weight of lugduname it would have the sweetness of 4500 kilograms (5000 tons) of sugar. That's the equivalent of two rhinos, or about 45 million bees (sticking with the honey theme).

ENDNOTES

1 Kellogg, J. H. *Plain facts for old and young: embracing the natural history and hygiene of organic life*. I.F. Segner (1887).

2 Clarkson, J. *Food History Almanac: Over 1,300 Years of World Culinary History, Culture, and Social Influence*. Rowman & Littlefield (2013).

3 Babu, R. The only taste: cyanide is acrid. *Hindustan Times* (8 July 2006). https://www.hindustantimes.com/india/the-only-taste-cyanide-is-acrid/story-vhsbYsiNyWzIfakN4HBK0H.html.

4 Nichols, C. Hitler's last food taster gets the novel treatment in bestseller 'At the Wolf's Table'. *ABC News* (4 April 2019). https://www.abc.net.au/news/2019-04-04/hitler-food-taster-novel-at-the-wolfs-table-rosella-postorino/10959950.

5 Rosenblum, I. et al. Single- and Double-Blind Studies with Oral Monosodium Glutamate in Man. *Toxicology and Applied Pharmacology*, 18 (2), 367–73 (1971).

VOICE (LOSS OF)

If you've ever lost your voice for even a few days, I'm sure you'd agree that life without a voice would be unspeakable.

Modern children are spoilt for choice when it comes to high-tech toys: voice-controlled racing cars, wi-fi-enabled robots, remote-controlled tanks that shoot rubber bullets. What happened to the good ol' days, when kids made their own fun with a stick or an oddly shaped rock? Let me cure you of that nostalgia. Practising in London in 1848, German physician Dr Karl August Burow became involved in an odd 'game' that the entertainment-starved local children had invented. His case report, published in 1850 in *The British and Foreign Medico-Chirurgical Review*, was titled: 'On the removal of the larynx [voice box] of a goose from that of a child by tracheostomy':

> The children in Dr. Burow's vicinity are very fond of blowing through the larynx of a recently-killed goose, in order to produce some imitation of the sound emitted by this animal ... A boy, aged 12, while so engaged (Nov. 1, 1848), was seized with a cough, and swallowed the instrument; a sense of suffocation immediately ensued, which was, after a while, replaced by great dyspnoea [trouble breathing].
>
> Dr. Burow found him labouring under this, eighteen hours after, his face swollen, of a bluish-red colour, and covered with perspiration. At every inspiration, the muscles of the

neck contracted spasmodically, and a clear, whistling sound was heard; and at each expiration, a hoarse sound, not very unlike that of a goose, was emitted. Tracheotomy [cutting a hole in the trachea] was at once performed; but owing to the homogeneousness of structure of the foreign body and of the parts it was in contact with, the greatest difficulty existed in distinguishing it by the forceps. At last, after repeated attempts, Dr. Burow having fixed the larynx in the neck by his forefinger ... he contrived to remove the entire larynx of the animal. The child was quite well by the ninth day.[1]

That's what happens when children don't have smartphones or Lego drones: one of the more curious ones will eventually get bored and inhale a goose's larynx.

*

Two tubes exit your mouth – the trachea in front for air, and the oesophagus behind for food. To avoid choking to death, it's important that food never enters the trachea. If a chunk of steak blocks your trachea then you can't get air in and out, a scenario that is 'not compatible with life' (as doctors euphemistically call any situation that will kill you). To prevent death-by-steak, a flap of gristle called the epiglottis seals off your trachea whenever you swallow. Saliva and steak simply slide over the epiglottis and slip back into the oesophagus. Between swallows your epiglottis sits up at a jaunty angle to allow air to flow in and out of your lungs.

Your larynx, commonly called the voice box, sits immediately beneath your epiglottis. It's a five-centimetre-long (two-inch-long) chamber that merges with the trachea at its base. Within this box lie your precious vocal cords.

Your Adam's apple is the knobbly facade to your voice box. Stroke the front of your neck and you should be able to discern this particularly prominent triangular protuberance (technically called the laryngeal prominence). Everyone has an Adam's apple, though it's usually more obvious in gents. Now, slide your fingers down until the point where your collar bones meet. You just stroked a length of your trachea. And it deserves a congratulatory pat: it's kept you alive and breathing all these years. The series of bumps you felt are the rings of cartilage that keep your trachea propped open. Your oesophagus has no need for such rings; between swallows, its slippery walls just collapse against each other. Your trachea, however, must permanently stay open what with your constant requirement to breathe.

Your two vocal cords are surprisingly soft and wet. Only a couple of centimetres (just under an inch) long, they're lined with the same slimy tissue as the inside of your cheek. Make a 'V-for-victory' or 'peace' sign with your fingers. With pleasing alphabetical appropriateness, this gesture nicely approximates the arrangement of your V-for vocal cords, with each finger acting as a cord. The base of the V faces forward and sits in your Adam's apple. The two V tips point towards your back. When you're silent, the cords rest about eight millimetres (0.31 inches) apart in this V shape (they have to be apart to let air pass down your trachea into your lungs). Bring your two fingers together, then apart. Your vocal cords close and open like this when you speak.

These two flimsy flaps let you talk, sing and shout from infancy until death. But how, exactly, does a pair of damp cords sitting in a box of gristle generate noise? For that, you need airflow.

Here's how it works. Blow up a balloon and pinch the neck closed. Holding the neck at the very edge, stretch it apart to slowly let some air out. You'll hear a noise as escaping air vibrates the neck of the deflating balloon. Your voice is produced in much the same way. The air reservoir is your lungs; the slapping edges of the balloon's neck are your vocal cords. When you exhale, the rush of air escaping your lungs vibrates your vocal cords as it passes through them. As the cords smack together some 100 to 1000 times per second the vibration produces a sound wave. You can only speak properly when exhaling: when you inhale, the cords have to adopt their separated V shape to let air in, hence no cord-slapping (noise generation) can occur. If you try to talk while inhaling, the best you'll manage is a sort of monotonous strangled sound that can be vaguely shaped into words.

The position your cords are in when they're vibrating affects the sound they'll produce. Your cords don't just open and shut; they're precisely lengthened, shortened, pulled apart and pushed together by ten tiny muscles attached to them. Tightly stretched cords produce higher-pitched sounds while looser cords produce lower-pitched notes, just like when tuning a violin string.

During puberty, testosterone enlarges the voice box and the cords within it. In both sexes, pre-pubescent vocal cords are about 17 millimetres (0.67 inches) long. Men, who produce more testosterone than women, end up with roomier voice boxes (which is why their Adam's apples usually jut out further) housing thicker, longer cords: about 29 millimetres (1.14 inches), a 70 per cent increase during puberty. Under testosterone's influence the cavities in men's noses, sinuses and back of the throat enlarge too. Chunkier cords plus more space for sound to resonate result in a deeper voice (think double bass compared to a violin). When a pubescent boy's voice 'breaks' – that period of embarrassing squeaks and unpredictable pitch changes – it's due to the laryngeal muscles learning to control the vocal cords as they (and their cartilaginous home) rapidly enlarge. Women's comparatively thinner, shorter vocal cords – reaching about 21 millimetres (0.83 inches), just a 24 per cent lengthening during puberty – vibrate faster than a man's (about 200 vibrations per second on average versus about 110 for men), hence women tend to have higher-pitched voices.

Testicles are a man's primary source of testosterone. If a boy is castrated before puberty, his voice box won't be flooded by the usual teenage testosterone tidal wave. As a result, his voice box will remain in its juvenile form forever. Clandestine castrations of young boys began in the 16th century to 'solve' the problem that women weren't allowed in stage productions or church choirs, yet someone needed to sing the soprano score. Since the surgery was illegal, the boy's missing testicles were usually attributed to some freak genital-focussed accident. When they grew up, these adult men housing child-sized voice boxes could generate a powerful, flexible voice with an unnaturally wide range, as unnatural as the cruel castration that gave them their abilities and their name, castrati. By the 18th century, the unique castrati voice was so revered that the majority of male opera singers were castrati. At the peak of the craze, it's estimated that some 4000 boys every year had their testicles removed in the hope of a successful career in the opera. Swiss-born composer and philosopher Jean-Jacques Rousseau lambasted this gruesome practice in his 1775 *Dictionary of Music*:

> In Italy there are barbarous fathers who sacrifice nature to money and permit their children to undergo this operation, merely to give pleasure to cruel voluptuaries who cultivate these poor creatures' voices.[2]

Thankfully the fad had largely died out by the start of the 19th century.

*

If all humans have the same vocal instrument – two vocal cords in a voice box – why are some people better singers than others? Well, some people are just born with an anatomical resonance chamber (their throat, mouth, and nasal cavities) whose dimensions yield better acoustics. But a crucial modifiable discriminator is vocal cord control. After all, a good singer is just someone who can reliably position their vocal cords to produce the note they want. Singing exercises, like scales and arpeggios, let your brain rehearse the sequence of muscle movements needed to tug your cords into the right position to create a particular sound. Of note, you can't strengthen your vocal cords any more than you can your ear lobes – they're not muscles. What vocal exercises strengthen is the communication between your brain and those ten cord-manipulating muscles. It's not all about the vocal cords either: you can boost your breath control by strengthening your diaphragm (which *is* a muscle) and tweaking your posture. With a bit of practice, anyone can sing!

Well, almost anyone.

About four per cent of the population have a condition called congenital amusia – tone deafness. Play them 'Happy Birthday' without lyrics and they won't recognise it. Ask them to identify a deliberate wrong note in 'Silent Night' and they'll stay silent. Tone deaf people can't recognise pitch, a skill that humans are usually born with. Babies usually wriggle more and look away from a speaker when it's playing dissonant tunes but sit still and stare mesmerised when in-tune music is playing. For the 96 per cent of people who aren't tone deaf, we just know – from birth – when a note isn't right.

Generating any sound requires the vibration of gas molecules to make a sound wave. When it comes to your voice, your vocal cords do the vibrating and the gas they vibrate is usually air. The air we breathe is a mixture of 21 per cent oxygen, 78 per cent nitrogen and one per cent other gases. But what would happen if your vocal cords vibrated a gas other than air? Lighter gas molecules like helium are zippier than the molecules in air. Helium-bathed vocal cords still vibrate at the same frequency, but the resulting sound waves travel three times faster through the helium than air. Demonstrations of the resulting squeaky voice invariably occur at any celebrations featuring alcohol and a supply of helium. Technically, helium doesn't make your voice take on a higher pitch, since pitch is the result of the frequency at which your cords vibrate. Instead, helium changes the timbre or tone of your voice. Conversely, inhaling a denser-than-air gas like sulfur hexafluoride (SF6) will give your voice a pleasingly deep timbre. SF6 is a potent greenhouse gas now largely banned from commercial use, but it used to be found in refrigerants and, until 2006, the 'air pockets' in the heels of Nike shoes.

*

What do teachers, colonels and football coaches have in common? They're all in charge of often unruly underlings who regularly need to be yelled at. To speak louder your lungs need to generate a stronger air current to blast your vocal cords wider apart. This stretches the cords, and results in a higher amplitude smack when they reunite. With repeated collisions your vocal cords can become inflamed, a condition called laryngitis. Infection with viruses or bacteria causes similar inflammation, which can involve the entire lining of your voice box. Stomach acid refluxing up your oesophagus (see *Acid reflux*, page 161) and spilling into your voice box can also cause laryngitis. Swollen, bloated cords move sluggishly and don't seal or vibrate properly. You experience this condition as a hoarse or lost voice. Your voice will be croaky until your cords' slimy lining heals and normal airflow control can resume.

People who repeatedly abuse their vocal cords – like those in the professions above – can develop nodules on their cords. These bumps prevent the cords closing properly, giving the voice a breathy, raspy Clint Eastwood-like quality. Surgery to remove the nodules is risky, since an over-zealous cut could scar and irreparably damage the cords. This was the fate of singer and actor, Julie Andrews, who filed a malpractice suit against her surgeons after she was left unable to sing following this surgery in 1997.

Permanent voice loss awaits those following a laryngectomy, the surgical removal of the voice box. Laryngeal cancer is the most common reason to have this procedure. About 95 per cent of people with laryngeal cancer are smokers. Cancer-causing chemicals in tobacco smoke mutate the cells lining the voice box. If you repeatedly infuse your voice box with puffs of carcinogenic smoke, one of those mutations might grow into a tumour.

Doctors standardise a person's smoking exposure by expressing it in 'pack-years'. If you've smoked one pack (twenty cigarettes) a day for 50 years, you have a 50 pack-year history of smoking. If you've smoked half a pack a day for 50 years, you have a 25 pack-year history of smoking. The longest history I've come across was a 65-year-old man with a 200 pack-year smoking history – that's five packs a day since age 15 (against all the odds, he didn't die from smoking-related cancer, but in a car crash). A 20 pack-year smoking history triples your risk of laryngeal cancer. A 40 pack-year history carries an eightfold risk.

Without vocal cords, a person who has had a laryngectomy has nothing left to vibrate to generate sound. Enter the electrolarynx: a vibrating device about the size of a Mars bar that jiggles the throat when pressed under the chin, providing the vibration that the vocal cords usually would. After many hours of training, the user can manipulate the artificial vibration using their tongue and lips into speech. Unfortunately, the resulting voice sounds robotic and unnatural: the device can never achieve the nuanced vibration that the finely controlled vocal cords can with their ten fancy muscles.

Since using an electrolarynx requires significant effort, and the resulting voice is hard to understand, why not transplant a voice box? Dead people can donate hearts and livers and kidneys: why not their larynxes too? Well, there are lots of reasons. From the surgeon's perspective, the neck is a minefield of crucial and complex structures like arteries and nerves. Operating in such an environment, a voice box transplant would be fiendishly fiddly and possibly lethal. Secondly, the recipient would be consigned to a life on heavy-duty medication to prevent their immune system rejecting the donated voice box. Thirdly, patients who require a laryngectomy to remove cancer generally have a limited lifespan; spending their remaining time on earth recovering from another major surgery is unlikely to be in their best interests, and the cancer might grow back in the transplant. Finally, the larynx is a non-vital organ, unlike a heart or liver. You can live without a voice box. It's ethically challenging to justify performing dangerous surgery that isn't strictly necessary.

For all those reasons, only a handful of voice box transplants have ever been performed. The first was conducted at the Cleveland Clinic in 1998, its outcome published in *The New England Journal of Medicine* accompanied by an editorial with the groan-worthy title: 'Transplantation of the Larynx – A Case Report That Speaks for Itself'.[3] The recipient was 40-year-old Tim Heidler. The day after his 21st birthday, Tim was motorbiking along a logging trail when he rode, neck-first, into a steel cable that had been strung between two trees. His throat was split open and his voice box irreparably damaged. For the next 20 years he relied on an electrolarynx to speak. Upon hearing that doctors were hunting for a patient to be the pioneering recipient of a voice box transplant, he immediately volunteered. Tim was an ideal transplant candidate: he lost his larynx from trauma, not cancer, and he was willing to accept the surgical risks and a subsequent life on medication. Three days after the operation, Tim uttered his first independent word in 20 years: 'hello'. Tim's quality of life improved immeasurably following his transplant. He reflected on life without a voice:

> Without communication, nothing works. That's why a lot of people who've had laryngectomies stay at home. They don't go out. They just sit at home and ferment to nothing. They're depressed.[4]

Tim was unemployed before his voice box transplant; post-op he became a motivational speaker.

SUMMARY: Exhaled air passing through your vocal cords causes them to vibrate and generate sound waves: the basis of your voice. If your vocal cords become inflamed by overuse or infection you lose your voice because swollen vocal cords can't vibrate normally.

AND ALSO ...

I say!

Notwithstanding the ethical and surgical challenges, imagine the joy of describing your garden's birdlife after receiving a voice box transplant from David Attenborough. Or of reading aloud post-transplant with the use of Stephen Fry's cords. Unfortunately, even if you could get their consent, such transplants would just give you a different voice, not the voice of those melodious men.

Like a good PR agent, all your vocal cords do is generate buzz. Your unique voice is the result of how this buzz travels and reverberates in your mouth, nose and sinuses. Think of how your voice changes when you have a blocked nose, for example. To 'transplant a voice' you'd need to perform an entire head transplant.

The shape and position of your soft palate, tongue and lips further modulates your voice. To demonstrate this, try saying 'kuh', 'tuh' and 'puh'. See how you needed to use each of those three structures, respectively, to make those sounds? As a child, you experimented with these movements and eventually learnt to produce the 44 speech sounds, called phonemes, needed to speak English. Greek has about half as many, while the Taa language, spoken by several thousand people in Namibia and Botswana, has more than 100 phonemes. If a particular phoneme doesn't exist in your native tongue (for English speakers, think of French's throaty 'r' in 'trois', or German's guttural 'ch' in 'Achtung!') your unaccustomed vocal apparatus might struggle to pronounce it.

Oh God, Adam's choking

The name Adam's apple is drawn from an interpretation of the Biblical tale in which Eve, driven by the serpent, goads

Adam into eating fruit from the 'hands-off' tree in the garden of Eden. The lump signifies the fruit of the tree passing down Adam's throat, acting as a permanent reminder of his misbehaviour. But food passes down the oesophagus, the tube behind the trachea, which means our Adam's apple is jutting out of the wrong tube. Further, the Bible never specifies that the forbidden fruit is an apple. Rather than squabble with ancient allegory, in 1895 anatomists introduced the neutral term 'laryngeal prominence' and swiftly moved on.

Why humans get choked up

The image of a wide-eyed lion choking on a gazelle is laughable. Actually, it's quite disturbing. But why is it that humans are prone to choking but a lion never does? Other animals like lions have distinctly separate tubes for air and food, while ours have a risky shared crossover point with just a flimsy trapdoor (the epiglottis) to keep food out of our lungs. Seemingly an evolutionary error, lowering the voice box from the back of the mouth down into the throat was crucial for developing speech. Rather than the vocal cords' vibrations simply exiting our lips as a grunt, now we had all that space in the back of our mouth to act as a modifying echo chamber. Plus, with the tongue now overlying the voice box, it could shape the airflow to create distinct noises – speech. While a shark may not choke to death on a seal, it certainly can't talk.

Before you get too choked up about your susceptibility to choking, spare a thought for lizards, who have an even more unfortunate evolutionary trade-off. A running lizard's body swings violently from side-to-side. While running, this movement means that air is shunted between the lungs rather than being exhaled and inhaled. In other words, lizards can't run and breathe at the same time. Watch a lizard lope and you'll notice it pausing periodically – it's not being pensive, it's just stopping to breathe.

Blowing your own trumpet

Speaking into a tube (like a toilet paper roll) deepens your voice because you've increased the length of tubing through which your voice can reverberate. The same applies to brass instruments. The tuba's lengthy 5.5-metre (18-foot) tubing produces its deep waddling-elephant sound. If you violently untwist a French horn (which you may be inclined to do if you've ever tried to learn it) it will stretch only 3.7 metres (12 feet), resulting in a higher-pitched sound. Brass players produce different notes by changing the shape of their lips or the length of piping through which their breath travels. Pressing a key on a brass instrument opens a detour circuit through which air is diverted. Air vibrating through longer tubing creates a deeper note.

Turning to nature, a bird's voice box sits at the base of its trachea, rather than perched on top of it like in humans. This arrangement means their voice box's vibrations travel through more tubing before leaving their beak, allowing birds to generate deep honking notes. Consider the trumpet manucode, a small bird whose dark, iridescent plumage makes it appear to have been doused in petrol. Its trachea, rather than being a straight tube, forms an absurdly long coiled slinky within its chest: six loops in total. This extra-long tubing allows it to produce an alarmingly deep, booming cry, as though it is indignant at having been doused in petrol. Incidentally, the trumpet manucode sounds nothing like a trumpet, adding to the list of misnomers in the brass section:

1. The French horn was invented by a German;
2. The euphonium produces thunderous, rich tones, yet its name means 'sweet-voiced';
3. Not all 'brass' instruments are made from brass (e.g. the alphorn is made of wood);
4. A woman's fallopian 'tubes' should be called fallopian *tubas*. Sixteenth century Italian anatomist Gabriele

Falloppio named these broad-ended pipes leading from ovary to uterus 'tubas' after their resemblance to the brass instrument. In Italian, the plural of 'tuba' is 'tube'. English readers misinterpreted this plural form to mean the English word 'tube', tacked on an 's', and Falloppio's tubas became 'tubes' evermore.

ENDNOTES

1   Periscope: Surgery. *British Foreign Medico-chirurgical Review*, 5 (9), 260–261 (1850).

2   Rousseau, J. J. *Complete Dictionary of Music: consisting of a copious explanation of all words necessary to a true knowledge and understanding of music.* Translated by Waring, W. AMS Press (1975).

3   Monaco, A. P. Transplantation of the Larynx–A Case Report That Speaks for Itself. *New England Journal of Medicine*, 344 (22), 1712–1714 (2001).

4   Whitley, M. A. Tim Heidler, world's first larynx transplant recipient at Cleveland Clinic, is doing well: Whatever happened to ...?. *Cleveland.com* (8 June 2009). https://www.cleveland.com/metro/2009/06/tim_heidler_worlds_first_laryn.html.

ACID REFLUX

How a low pH fluid causes sky-high pain.

In June 1822, 18-year-old Alexis St. Martin was working as a boat porter for the American Fur Company. He spent his days paddling hunters around North America's waterways as they shot various fluffy mammals. On June 6, St. Martin was killing time between rowing jobs in a shop on Mackinac Island in Michigan's Lake Huron. A clumsy duck hunter entered the store holding a loaded musket. He sidled up to St. Martin and, at a close range, accidentally fired a round straight into St. Martin's stomach. The explosion of gunpowder and lead shot created 'a perforation ... directly into the cavity of the stomach'.[1]

That quote is courtesy of Dr William Beaumont, a 27-year-old US Army surgeon stationed nearby who was called to attend to St. Martin:

> I saw him in twenty-five or thirty minutes after the accident occurred, and, on examination, found a portion of the lung as large as a turkey's egg, protruding through the external wound, lacerated and burnt; and immediately below this, another protrusion, which, on further examination, proved to be a portion of the stomach ... pouring out the food he had taken for his breakfast, through an orifice large enough to admit the forefinger.

Beaumont provided first aid and took St. Martin in under his care. At first, any food that St. Martin swallowed just spewed from the wound. Beaumont noted: 'the only way of sustaining him was via nutritious injections per rectum.' After 17 days, food would finally remain in his stomach if the gunshot wound was plugged with cloth. Once the wound had healed, St. Martin was left with a fistula: a neat hole in the skin 'about the size of a shilling piece' leading directly to his stomach. Beaumont smelt an opportunity:

> This case affords a most excellent opportunity of experimenting upon the gastric fluids, and the process of digestion. It would give no pain, nor cause the least uneasiness, to extract a gill of fluid every two or three days, for it frequently flows out spontaneously in considerable quantities; and one might introduce various digestible substances into the stomach, and easily examine them during the whole process of digestion.[2]

Many of Beaumont's experiments (there were 238 of them) involved examining the contents of St. Martin's stomach at intervals after he had eaten a meal. Not all the meals were swallowed. Sometimes Beaumont would fill a drawstring muslin bag with food and poke it directly through the fistula into St. Martin's stomach. He would periodically fish the bag out via the dangling silk string to check on the digestive process. St. Martin apparently 'complained of some pain and uneasiness at the breast' during this procedure. The test menu was extensive, including items as disparate as 'recently salted lean beef', 'eight ounces of calf's foot jelly', 'three ripe apples', and 'raw oysters'. Every few hours after ingestion, St. Martin's stomach contents would be examined. For example:

> At 8 o'clock, 30 minutes, A.M. [St. Martin] breakfasted on bread and butter and one pint of coffee. 9 o'clock 45 minutes, examined; stomach full of fluids. 10 o'clock, examined;

and took out a portion resembling thin gruel in colour and consistence [sic], with the oil of the butter floating on the top, a few small particles of the bread and some mucus falling to the bottom; about two-thirds digested. It had a sharp acid taste.[1]

Yes, Beaumont routinely tasted St. Martin's stomach contents and documented his findings:

Experiment 11: at 10 o'clock P.M, after eighteen hours' fasting, introduced tube and drew off one and a half hours of gastric juice. It was clear, and almost transparent; tasted a little saltish and acid when applied to the tongue.

Harvested samples of stomach juices were used to 'digest' food in cups. This dispelled the long-standing belief that digestion was a mechanical effect of stomach churning: in fact, it was predominantly a chemical process performed by stomach acid. Beaumont discovered that 'severe exercise' resulted in 'retarded digestion' and also commented on the size and shape of the stomach:

When entirely empty, [St. Martin's] stomach contracts upon itself, and sometimes forces [through the fistula] and forms a tumour as large as a hen's egg.

Beaumont seemed to have a penchant for describing objects in terms of specific birds' eggs.

Initially, St. Martin was grateful for Beaumont's life-saving care and complied with his fanciful experiments. But after ten years of off-and-on experimentation, the novelty had worn off. In 1832 Beaumont had the illiterate St. Martin sign a contract requiring him, in return for a small allowance and board, to submit to 'the exhibiting and showing of his stomach' plus any 'physiological or medical experiments as [Beaumont] shall direct or cause to be made on or in the stomach of him'.[3]

The pair parted ways in 1834. St. Martin died in 1880 from a head injury after slipping on thin ice, an appropriate metaphor for the ethically precarious partnership he had endured with Beaumont.

*

St. Martin was shot in his stomach. Point to where you think his bullet wound was. Wrong! Well, you may have guessed correctly, but I suspect you were pointing somewhere in the vicinity of your belly button. St. Martin's wound was actually about five centimetres (two inches) below his left nipple. That's right, your stomach sits beneath your left-sided ribs. In the mirror-image position under your right-sided ribs is your liver. To reiterate – both organs sit high up *under your ribs*. Continuing with the tour around the abdomen, your spleen is wedged on the far left next to your stomach. Peep behind your stomach and you'll spot your pancreas, draped like a warty yellow slug across your vertebrae. Your kidneys also sit against your back on either side of the spine, largely protected within your rib cage. The take-home message is that many of your abdominal organs are positioned much higher than you probably thought, safeguarded by your ribcage. The soft exposed hinterland where you thought your stomach sat is largely occupied by your 7.5 metres (25 feet) of intestines (see *Diarrhoea*, page 194).

Every day your stomach produces two litres (half a gallon) of gastric juice, a clear liquid that is mainly water plus electrolytes, like sodium and potassium, enzymes (chemicals that assist with digestion) and, most importantly, hydrochloric acid. The acidity of gastric juice is very useful. Acid kills microbes in your meals, breaks down tough chunks of food that you were too lazy to chew properly, and helps you absorb certain vitamins like calcium, B12 and iron.

Vultures can eat putrid roadkill without suffering food poisoning thanks to their immensely corrosive stomach acid – 10 to 100 times more acidic than yours. At that extreme acidity, the bugs responsible for botulism, anthrax, cholera and rabies just fizzle up and die if they happen to be ingested. At the other end of the spectrum, anteaters don't even bother to make stomach acid. They just let swallowed ants digest in their own formic acid, released when the anteater munches on them.

To safeguard against acidic autodigestion, your stomach's walls are smeared with a thick alkaline gel. The cells that make up your stomach's lining are tightly sealed like a wall of bricks and mortar to prevent acid leaks. This mucous-lined, no-gap barrier means you can eat and digest a cow's stomach (as in tripe) but you won't digest your own. Equally, you could eat and digest another human's stomach, but you may be arrested.

Between meals, your gastric juice's pH can drop to 1 – only slightly less acidic than battery acid. If you dripped gastric juice on your arm, your skin would dissolve. When you eat, the food and saliva entering your stomach dilutes your stomach juices and brings the pH up to about 4 (the pH of acid rain, or tomato juice).

Your savvy stomach has a few ways to ramp up its acid production to return its juice's pH to a more effective acidity. First is the pre-emptive strategy: smelling, seeing or merely thinking about food stimulates gastric acid production. Next, when food enters your stomach, cells in the stomach wall called 'G cells' respond by releasing a hormone called gastrin (the G in G-cell stands for gastrin: science isn't always complicated). Gastrin tells your stomach's acid-producing glands to squirt out more acid. Finally, as your stomach stretches to accommodate your meal, it releases further gastrin. And your stomach can really stretch. From its empty volume of 80 millilitres (the size of a duck's egg, as Beaumont might say), it can expand 50-fold to accommodate a mind boggling four litres (one gallon) and protrude all the way into your pelvis.

While your stomach may be acid-proof, the rest of your gut is not. Food typically marinates in the acid bath of your stomach for about four hours. Waves of muscular contractions churn the food to assist its breakdown into a mush called chyme. The stomach empties this acidic chyme into your small intestine, the first part of which is called the duodenum (from the Greek *dodekadaktylon* meaning twelve fingers long, because it is). Chyme's acidity 'presents a tremendous challenge' for the duodenum, as eloquently stated by the authors of the 1987 paper 'Alkaline Secretion'.[4] As you may have guessed from the paper's title, the duodenum protects itself from acid burns by producing an alkaline secretion: a basic mucous. Basic in both senses of the word: it's alkaline, and it's simple – just mucous and bicarbonate. This provides your duodenum with a protective coating much like that in the stomach. But your gastrointestinal tract can't be expected to keep making gallons of protective mucous all the way to your anus. The chyme needs to be rendered neutral.

Thankfully, when chyme hits your duodenum it's met with a wave of alkaline juices courtesy of your pancreas. A garnish of bile (pH 8), provided by your gallbladder, provides another natural antacid. Both of these fluids enter your duodenum via a muscular ring buried in its wall, named the sphincter of Oddi.[*] Upon mixing with these alkaline fluids, chyme's pH rises from a gut-perforating 2 to an intestinally innocuous 6. Now neutralised, your semi-digested food can pass through the rest of your gut without burning holes in it.

*

To reach your stomach, your food must travel through your chest and diaphragm. The food's conveyor tube – your oesophagus – runs behind your heart and lungs, just in front of your spinal column. And I mean 'just in front': your oesophagus literally sits flat against your spine next to your aorta. If you fracture your

---

[*] Its Italian discoverer, Ruggero Oddi (1864–1913), was stood down as director of the Physiological Institute of Genoa in 1900 due to 'fiscal improprieties' and odd behaviour stemming from recreational narcotic use.

upper vertebrae you run the risk of your oesophagus being ripped open by bone shards. Having traversed the chest, your oesophagus passes through a hole in your diaphragm and joins the saggy sac of your stomach. The journey from your teeth to your stomach is about 40 centimetres (16 inches).

Hydrochloric acid is terrific for cleaning bricks. But your oesophagus isn't a brick that needs cleaning. Instead, it's a 30-centimetre-long (12-inch-long) muscular tube with a slimy delicate lining. Ideally, stomach acid should stay in the stomach. If it sloshes up into the lower oesophagus, it hurts. The pain is typically an ascending burning pain, as though acid were rising through your chest – because it is.

Despite being called heartburn, the pain of acid reflux has nothing to do with your heart. But the misnomer is understandable since the pain of a heart attack and heartburn can feel very similar: a burning sensation behind the breastbone. It's important to distinguish between the two, as they have rather different treatments. When faced with a patient clutching their chest in agony, ever-practical emergency doctors often perform a quick experiment: they get the patient to swallow a shot of local anaesthetic mixed with antacid. If the patient is experiencing acid reflux, this cocktail numbs their acid-burnt oesophagus and the pain disappears. If the patient is having a heart attack however, the pain will persist.

In your body, any muscular ring that controls fluid flow is called a sphincter. I recently introduced you to your sphincter of Oddi. You might be familiar with your anal sphincters (yes, you've got more than one: see *Farts and burps*, page 207) which keep faeces and farts from falling out of you at random. Your urethral sphincter does the same for urine. Innumerable sphincters in your blood vessels divert and reroute blood throughout your body. When it comes to preventing reflux, it's the lower oesophageal sphincter that does the job. This ring of muscle at the base of your oesophagus, wrapped just above where it joins your stomach, keeps the lower oesophagus pinched closed between swallows. You can do a cartwheel or stand on your head, and it will throttle your oesophagus tightly enough to keep your stomach juices in place. Having a lower oesophageal sphincter means that stomach acid containment doesn't rely on gravity, hence astronauts who dine upside down are no more prone to getting reflux than us earthlings.

Reflux is the result of a malfunctioning lower oesophageal sphincter that allows stomach juices to splash up into your oesophagus.

You've got no control over your lower oesophageal sphincter: it's an involuntary muscle just like the ones that squeeze food through your intestines. You can't will it to squeeze harder or strengthen it with training. Some people just have a weak sphincter that makes them prone to reflux. But most sphincters become slack due to something else. Smoking and alcohol don't just relax your mind: they also relax your lower oesophageal sphincter. Some medications used to treat high blood pressure work by dilating your blood vessels to decrease the pressure in your arteries. Their dilating effects can extend to your lower oesophageal sphincter too. Fatty foods have been shown to relax the lower oesophageal sphincter. Not by literally greasing it, but by triggering chemical pathways that affect muscle function. Chocolate and peppermint have a similar effect.

Patients with reflux are told to avoid spicy foods. This isn't because those foods cause reflux, but because refluxed fluid containing chilli really hurts when it splashes your already acid-burned lower oesophagus.

High internal stomach pressures can overcome the lower oesophageal sphincter's squeezing capacity. Upward pressure from a stuffed stomach after a large meal can cause 'vomit burps': bubbles of gastric contents that break through the sphincter's iron grip. Anything that increases abdominal pressure – a pregnant uterus, excess fat, wearing a corset – can cause reflux via similar upward forces that blow open the sphincter. Even brief pressure increases from coughing, bending over or straining on the toilet can be enough to bust open that sphincter.

*

Acid reflux isn't just painful: it can cause serious oesophageal damage. Acid can erode the lining of your oesophagus and form ulcers. Healed ulcers form stiff scars that can create oesophageal narrowings called strictures. If a stricture is very tight, food might get stuck en route to the stomach and result in choking. Particularly forceful sprays of refluxing acid can reach the back of the throat. It can then spill into the voice box and cause chronic laryngitis, or trickle down the trachea and cause a persistent cough (see *Cough*, page 167).

Your body is skilled at adapting to repeated harmful stimuli. If you take up barefoot walking, the skin on the soles of your feet will soon thicken into protective callouses. If you lift a pair of dumbbells, you'll tear some of the muscle fibres in your biceps. They'll respond to the injury by fusing into larger, stronger muscle fibres. This is how weight-lifting bulks up your muscles: via repeated cycles of deliberate muscle tearing and healing. Your oesophagus can also adapt to repeated damage from acid reflux. Its solution is to transform those acid-splashed cells at its base into more acid-resistant cells. The same sort of acid-resistant cells, in fact, that line your stomach. If you put a camera down an oesophagus that has undergone this adaptation, its lower end looks identical to the stomach – deep red – rather than its usual salmon-pink. We call this condition Barrett's oesophagus, after Australian-born surgeon Norman Barrett who first described it in 1950. Barrett mistakenly thought that what he was looking at was a bit of herniated stomach trapped in the chest, rather than a mutated oesophageal lining.

Although this acid-proofing adaptation seems useful, the problem is that when cells mutate, they don't always stop mutating. Cells that mutate out of control form tumours. People with Barrett's oesophagus have a 30-fold increased risk of developing oesophageal cancer. To prevent Barrett's oesophagus and the associated cancer risk, it's important that people with reflux take medication to reduce the amount of acid their stomach makes. If the contents of the refluxed fluid are less acidic, the cells lining the lower oesophagus are less likely to sustain damage and mutate in response.

Humans with acid reflux undoubtedly experience pain and suffering. But spare a thought for the giant squid, whose oesophagus travels through a hole in the middle of its brain. The squid has to rip its food into tiny morsels to prevent brain damage from swallowing a piece of prawn too big to squeeze through its brain hole. If we get acid reflux we just feel heartburn, but a poor giant squid with reflux must experience brainburn.

SUMMARY: Your stomach is filled with acidic juice which is important for killing swallowed microbes and digesting your food. But if the juice sloshes through a malfunctioning lower oesophageal sphincter, its acidity burns your oesophageal lining and causes pain.

AND ALSO ...

Why surgeons are fast to ask you to fast

Surgeries tend to be more successful when the patient is unconscious and still. For this reason, a general anaesthetic contains muscle relaxants as well as drugs that knock you unconscious. With your breathing muscles disabled, you need a tube down your throat attached to a machine that breathes for you. Your floppy limbs are carefully secured to the table by padded straps. Your lower oesophageal sphincter also relaxes, making reflux almost inevitable. Since you're paralysed, you can't cough like you usually would if the refluxed stomach contents drip into your trachea. Notwithstanding the acid burns to your airways, an inhaled chunk of that morning's toast might block off part of your lung and will almost certainly become infected. This is why you're told to fast before an operation: being anaesthetised on an empty stomach ensures that when you inevitably regurgitate, at least it'll only be a very small volume of juice (and certainly no bits of food).

An expensive (and expansive) way to die

Acid reflux causes an ascending burning pain in your chest. But the corresponding descending burning pain can be achieved by pouring liquid gold or other molten metals down the throat. This gruesome form of execution was once meted out by the Romans, Native Indians of the Jivaro tribe, and Spanish Inquisitors among others. But by what precise mechanism would it kill you? Researchers in 2003 sought to find out.[5] Due to budgetary constraints, in lieu of gold they used 750 grams (26 ounces) of lead. Moral scruples have improved since the Spanish Inquisition, so rather than using a live heretic, they experimented with the upper airway of a slaughtered cow. Upon pouring molten lead – at 450°C (842°F) – into the disembodied throat of the cow, massive jets of steam spurted from either end. The scientists concluded that it was steam pressure that likely over-inflated and burst open the heretic's lungs, swiftly resulting in death via steam implosion. Plus, they helpfully pointed out, the molten metal when solidified would block the voice box and suffocate the victim, if the steam-rupturing hadn't done the trick.

A tad uncomfortable

Reflux is uncomfortable, but it's nothing like the pain of childbirth. Unless you're a gastric-brooding frog, whose method of tadpole delivery was regurgitation. These frogs are now extinct, presumably due to this ridiculously unsustainable method of reproduction. The female would lay her eggs, wait for a male to fertilise them, then swallow the fertilised eggs whole. The jelly halo surrounding each egg contained a chemical that switched off her stomach's acid production. Unfortunately, the chemical took a while to kick in, so the mother frog would digest the first half of the eggs she swallowed. Her makeshift stomach-womb would expand over the following six weeks as the tadpoles hatched and matured (their gill mucous continuing to keep her stomach acid at bay). Eventually she would regurgitate each fully formed froglet one at a time over several days. If startled, she would unceremoniously regurgitate her brood all at once, an event no doubt uncomfortable for all parties involved.

ENDNOTES

1   Beaumont, W. *Experiments and Observations on the Gastric Juice, and the Physiology of Digestion.* MacLachlan & Stewart (1838).

2   Webster, J. A Case of Wounded Stomach. *The Medical Recorder,* 8 (1825).

3   Horsman, R. *Frontier Doctor: William Beaumont, America's First Great Medical Scientist.* University of Missouri Press (1996).

4   Wenzl, E., et al. Alkaline secretion. *Gastroenterology,* 92 (3), 709–715 (1987).

5   van de Goot, F. R. W. Molten gold was poured down his throat until his bowels burst. *Journal of Clinical Pathology,* 56 (2), 157 (2003).

COUGH

'Love and a cough cannot be hid.'
George Herbert

Hospital patients with productive coughs are provided with a container called a sputum mug. On one memorable night shift, I was paged to review a delirious elderly woman with pneumonia. Upon my arrival I saw her sipping a cup of tea. In the sickening moment when I realised that she had confused her tea mug with her sputum mug I knew that I could never become a respiratory physician; or eat mayonnaise again.

Mucous coats your airways and nostrils. Every day, your lungs make about a tablespoon of mucous to trap the detritus floating in the 11,000-odd litres (2900 gallons) of air you inhale. An escalator of microscopic hairs called cilia (pronounced 'sillier') constantly swishes the mucous from the depths of your airways towards the back of your throat for you to swallow or cough up. Each cell lining your nose and throat has about 200 cilia which beat 10 to 20 times per second. Cilia can also be found in a woman's fallopian tubes (or should I say fallopian *tubas*: see *Voice (loss of)*, page 151) to beat an ovulated egg towards her uterus, and in a man's testicles to swoosh out his sperm.

Your cilia keep doggedly beating even when you're dead. They're the last part of you to stop moving, taking up to 20 hours to finally become still. They slow down at a predictable rate before they finally stop. Crime scene pathologists examining a fresh corpse can measure the beating rate of nasal cilia to estimate the time of death. This is more accurate than any decline in body temperature, which can be affected by the weather and clothing. If a corpse is found in a burnt-out building, airway examination can also provide vital clues to suggest foul-play. If the victim's airways are filled with soot and charred cilia, it suggests that they were alive and breathing while the fire was raging. We can conclude that the fire probably killed them. But if their airways are soot-free, with cilia intact, then they must have already stopped breathing when the fire was lit. It wasn't the fire that killed them: instead, the inferno may have been lit by the murderer to dispose of the corpse.

When your airways are infected, your immune system ramps up mucous production. Slime-entombed bugs can't replicate or invade. Incidentally, The Blob – the alien in the 1958 sci-fi movie starring Steve McQueen – employed a similar technique by engulfing humans. Phlegm and sputum are exchangeable terms for the thick mucous generated deep in your lungs, as distinct from the watery mucous that drips from your nose. Mucous-making cells are called goblet cells after their wine-goblet shape. Why respiratory physicians insist on associating mucous with drinking receptacles like mugs and goblets is beyond me. As infection sets in, the goblet cells in your airways increase in size, number, and volume of mucous production. Cilia sweep the globs of phlegm, in which microbes are suspended, towards the back of your throat for you to hack up into a mug (or goblet) or swallow, whereupon the bugs die in the acid bath of your stomach. Some ingenious bacteria like *Bordetella pertussis** (which causes whooping cough) release toxins that paralyse your cilia, thwarting phlegm clearance.

Coughing is your lungs' basic defence mechanism. The forceful gush of air rips microbe-filled mucous off the walls of your airways

---

* *Bordetella* is named after Jules Bordet (1870-1961), the Belgian microbiologist who discovered the bacteria in 1906. Pertussis means 'extremely cough' from the Latin *per* and *tussis*.

and sprays them into your environment. Countless viruses and bacteria can be rocketed out in this unappealing mist. When you've got an airway infection, these regular evacuations decimate the microbial colonies in your lungs, reducing the number of bugs that your immune system has to eliminate. Coughing also can dislodge inhaled foreign objects. During a 1924 expedition climbing Mount Everest, British mountaineer and surgeon Howard Somervell suddenly started choking. He gasped and coughed prodigiously, finally ejecting the obstruction. On close inspection, it turned out to be the frostbitten lining of his larynx. The dead, frozen chunk of flesh had dislodged and momentarily plugged his trachea.

Trying to quell a cough is fruitless, particularly when a frozen larynx is stuck in your throat. This is because coughing is a reflex – an action that your body performs without your conscious control. Other reflexes are sneezing, blinking when a projectile approaches your eye, and vomiting a bit into your mouth when a patient shows you the contents of their sputum mug. Your cough reflex is activated when cough receptors – super-sensitive nerve endings in your airways – are triggered, physically or chemically. Physical triggers can be trivial, like the featherlight pressure from inhaling the cocoa dust atop a cappuccino or hot chocolate. More ominously, pressure from a growing lung tumour can set them off too. Chemical cough triggers include inhaled smoke, chlorine gas, and violently refluxed stomach contents that make it into your airways. Studies in guinea pigs show that very salty liquids and capsaicin, the chemical that puts the heat into chillies, can also reliably trigger cough.

Once activated, cough receptors shoot off a message to your brainstem via a nerve called the vagus nerve. The nerve's name comes from the Latin for 'wandering', after its circuitous path around your organs. If you traced the vagus nerve's vagrant course from your brainstem, you'd see its branches wander through your ears, around your heart, oesophagus and into your guts. Vagus nerve activation at any of these locations can trigger your cough reflex. Wax-impaction or an ear hair tickling your eardrum can make you cough by triggering the vagus nerve's branch to the ear (known as Arnold's nerve,* the resulting cough referred to as 'Arnold's nerve ear-cough reflex'). Cough can result from an inflamed heart lining, or even mild acid reflux (the acid doesn't have to slosh into your airways to make you cough; just splashing the vagus nerve's lower oesophageal branches can set you spluttering).

Once your brainstem receives the vagus nerve's message that cough receptors have been activated, there's no turning back. Coordinated by your brainstem (not your brain: remember, you have no conscious control over coughing), first you take in a large gasp of air as your chest expands and your diaphragm pushes your guts down, sucking air into your lungs via negative pressure. To trap the air, your vocal cords and epiglottis – the gristly flap overlying your trachea – snap shut. Next, your abs and chest wall muscles contract, forcing your guts back up and squashing your lungs under your ribs. This compresses the air trapped in your lungs into a much smaller space, creating sky-high pressure. Finally, your vocal cords and epiglottis burst open to release the pent-up air at speeds approaching 80 kilometres (50 miles) per hour. As air rips through your airways faster than a greyhound it makes a fittingly bark-like sound – a cough.

A cough too weak to dislodge inhaled food can be deadly. Recall that stage one of coughing is deep inhalation. If you've got a hunk of steak blocking your trachea, this is impossible. First aid advice in a choking situation is to 'encourage the person to cough', then after they shoot you an exasperated glare indicating 'what do you think I'm trying to do?!', slap them five times between the shoulder blades. If that fails, perform the Heimlich manoeuvre five times: standing behind them, make a fist above their bellybutton, grab it with your other hand then press in and up, hard. Forty-two years after he created the eponymous

---

* Friedrich Arnold (1803–1890), an anatomy professor at Heidelberg who traced the vagus nerve's vagrant course from the brainstem of cadavers.

manoeuvre, a 96-year-old Dr Henry Heimlich employed his technique to save a choking nursing home co-resident. Alas, the Heimlich manoeuvre only works if there's a good Samaritan around to perform it. Every New Year, a handful of Japanese people die after choking on glutinous rice cakes called mochi. Authorities release annual public service announcements warning that mochi should be chewed carefully and 'never be eaten alone'. Choking to death on mochi, on a lonely New Year's Eve without a friend to save you, must surely be one of the most depressing ways to die.

*

It's long been claimed that an astute doctor can diagnose a cough based on its sound. Medical texts insist on printing these archaic, useless descriptions, which I will perpetuate here if only to deride them. A 'barking seal-like' cough typifies croup (a viral infection of the upper airway). A honking cough reminiscent of a Canada goose is seen in tic disorders like Tourette syndrome. A 'staccato cough' in an infant suggests a *Chlamydial* lung infection (*Chlamydia* bacteria don't just infect genitals). An inspiratory 'whoop' *can* accompany *Bordetella pertussis* infection, though in half of patients there's no big whoop. These outdated descriptions are rarely helpful. I'm yet to hear any doctor exclaim: 'Hark! The honk of a Canada goose! Prithee, take me to thy tic-disordered patient!' Instead, the most useful practical cough distinction is dry versus wet (or productive).

Dry coughs are usually due to a viral upper airway infection with one of the hundred or so rhinoviruses that cause the common cold. Inhaled viruses enter the cells lining your airways, hijack the cell's resources to replicate, then burst out. They kill the cell in the process before infecting its neighbour. Cell by cell, the trachea's lining erodes to reveal the cough receptors beneath. Exposed, the receptors now twitchily activate at the slightest stimulation.

Pressure from inflammation-driven swelling triggers even more coughing, as does the chemical soup secreted by the viruses, your immune response and dying cells.

Wet coughs are always abnormal. Something must be driving the excess mucous production, be it infection, a foreign body or chronic inflammation. It's a myth that eating dairy will increase mucous levels when you've got a productive cough. It's not as if yoghurt's similarly creamy consistency will inspire your goblet cells to ramp up production.

Doctors are trained to enquire about the colour of patients' phlegm. I never really want to know the answer, but I'm contractually obliged to ask. Neutrophils are 'white' blood cells that are actually faintly green due to the pigment myeloperoxidase. Neutrophils are heavily involved in fighting airway infections. Shortly after being infected, before your immune system has time to recruit neutrophils, your phlegm will be clear. When neutrophils rock up in modest numbers your phlegm will turn light green, usually perceived as yellow when mixed in shiny mucous. As infection progresses the neutrophil concentration reaches a peak: more concentrated myeloperoxidase renders your phlegm truly green. Neutrophils respond to both viral and bacterial infections. Having yellow or green phlegm just suggests infection; it gives no indication as to whether or not antibiotics (which only kill bacteria) are required.

Other phlegm colours give doctors diagnostic hints too. Bleeding airways, unsurprisingly, turn phlegm red. Usually the bleeding is from minor airway erosion during infection, but can suggest a more serious cause (such as a lung cancer that has eaten into a deep blood vessel, or a growing ball of tuberculosis bacteria). Tar from heavy smoking turns phlegm black or brown. Creamy white phlegm suggests persistent airway inflammation without infection (like asthma, or chronic obstructive pulmonary disease). Here, neutrophils are absent (so no green) but the inflammation attracts other white blood cells that cloud up the usually clear mucous. Purple, orange and blue phlegm can be seen in saliva-contaminated samples from patients who have recently eaten icy-poles of the same colour (a genuine confusion in paediatric wards where icy-poles are used as bribes to make children agree to having blood tests).

Inhaling various dusts can result in a host of lung diseases. The dust lodges deep in the lungs, causing inflammation resulting in coughing, trouble breathing and lung scarring. Many of these diseases are related to specific exposures, and are thusly named:

- bird fancier's lung (inhaling bird droppings and feathers)
- cheese washer's lung (mouldy cheese rinds)
- farmer's lung (mouldy hay)
- hot tub lung (microbe-filled steam)
- soy sauce lung (fermentation starter for soy sauce)
- mushroom worker's lung (mushroom compost)
- and the ridiculously specific: Japanese summer house lung (damp mats and wood).

The term 'bagpipe lung' was coined in 2016 after a 61-year-old bagpiper died from lung disease caused by fungi lurking in his bagpipes. His medical history held a vital clue: his symptoms rapidly improved when he abandoned his bagpipes during a three-month holiday in Australia. When he returned to the UK and resumed playing, his breathing deteriorated rapidly. Chasing this clue, doctors swabbed the instrument's mouthpiece and damp internal bag. A host of fungi were identified, the spores of which the bagpiper had been inhaling every time he played.

Rare fungal diseases aside, professional musicians generally have healthy lungs. The same cannot be said of their audience members. Attend any classical music concert and you may wonder if you've accidentally crashed a matinée for the local hospital's respiratory ward. The Austrian concert pianist Alfred Brendel once famously threatened his audience: 'Either you stop coughing or I stop playing.' In a 2012 paper, German academic Andreas Wagener applied behavioural economic principles in an attempt to explain the phenomenon of 'concert cough':

Concert etiquette demands that audiences of classical concerts avoid inept noises such as coughs. Yet, coughing in concerts occurs more frequently than elsewhere, implying a widespread and intentional breach of concert etiquette.[1]

Wagener concluded that 'coughing in concerts is excessive and non-random'. The average concertgoer coughs 0.025 times per minute, implying 36 coughs per person per day – far more than double the usual frequency. Coughing isn't evenly distributed throughout the performance either: it escalates during quieter, slower movements. Wagener suggested that coughing allows 'participation' in the concert in an effort to 'convey prestige and status, allow for demarcation and inclusion, produce conformity, and affirm individual and social values'.

SUMMARY: A cough is a reflex that jettisons foreign material from your lungs. These might be big things (mochi) or small things (like bacteria suspended in a glob of mucous). Coughing keeps your lungs clear of everything but air.

AND ALSO ...

A hacking cough – the cliché of writing hacks

Chekhov's Gun is a principle in drama that anything superfluous to a story's plot should be removed. The Russian writer Anton Chekhov was clear in his view: 'If in the first act you have hung a pistol on the wall, then in the following one it should be fired. Otherwise don't put it there.' Cough is the medical version of Chekhov's Gun: a coughing character must die. Alexander Dumas, fils (French for son), first popularised the 'coughing tragic heroine' trope in his 1852 novel *La Dame aux Camélias*. Marguerite starts coughing in Chapter 9:

> Toward the end of supper Marguerite was seized by a more violent fit of coughing than any she had had while I was there. It seemed as if her chest were being torn in two. The poor girl turned crimson, closed her eyes under the pain, and put her napkin to her lips. It was stained with a drop of blood.

Marguerite dies 17 chapters later. Plagues of pale women clutching lace-edged handkerchiefs have subsequently coughed and died their way through literary history: Mimì in Puccini's *La Bohème* (in Act 3, Mimì has 'a terrible cough' that 'shakes her weak frame', then dies in Act 4), Fantine in Victor Hugo's *Les Misérables* (she dismisses her 'little cough' but is dead by the end of Act 1), Helen in Charlotte Brontë's *Jane Eyre* (in Chapter 8, Helen 'breathed a little fast and coughed a short cough'. She dies in Chapter 9).

The implication is that each character has tuberculosis. Coughing up blood, night sweats and weight loss (hence the synonym 'consumption' – the disease consumes the energy stored in your muscle and fat (see *Fever*, page 42) – are the tell-tale signs. To be fair, in the 19th century tuberculosis caused a quarter of all deaths in Europe, so it was a natural go-to for authors.

ENDNOTES

1 Wagener, A. Why do people (not) cough in concerts: the economics of concert etiquette. *ACEI Working Paper Series* (2012).

GUTS

NAUSEA AND VOMITING

Why your brain thinks that it's saving your life by making you spew at sea.

Astronauts prepare for life in zero gravity by training in reduced-gravity aircraft. These planes give astronauts a taste of weightlessness and often a taste of their own vomit, hence their ominous nickname: vomit comets. The aircraft don't leave Earth's atmosphere, but their parabolic flight path – repeated 45-degree ascents and nosedives – can achieve brief periods of weightlessness. Each parabola lasts 65 seconds with about 25 seconds of floating time. If you thought sitting through one parabola sounded bad enough, a training flight typically involves 30 to 40 of these stomach-churning manoeuvres. John Yaniec, former lead test director of NASA's Reduced Gravity Program, claimed that vomit comet passengers felt queasy according to: 'a rule of thirds – one third violently ill, the next third moderately ill, and the final third not at all'.[1] Since Yaniec's job required him to sit through over 31,000 parabolas, it's lucky that he counted himself among that final third.

Despite vomit comet training, during their first days in orbit about 70 per cent of astronauts suffer some degree of space sickness or space adaptation syndrome as it's technically known. Without the pull of gravity, astronauts enter a nauseating topsy-turvy world where up and down don't exist. Space sickness came to the fore in 1961 when Soviet cosmonaut Gherman Titov, the second man to orbit the earth, became the first human to spew in space. When his capsule *Vostok-2* detached from its booster, plunging Titov into weightlessness, he experienced an illusion of cartwheeling: 'I felt suddenly as though I were turning a somersault and then flying with my legs up.' A few Earth orbits later, he vomited.

In addition to up/down confusion, astronauts can experience the illusion of missing limbs. Your muscles, joints and tendons contain receptors that detect stretch: how taut your bicep is, for example, or what angle your elbow is bent at. Your brain uses stretch receptor feedback to maintain a mental map of where your limbs are, without you having to look. This ability, called proprioception, allows you to walk without watching your feet or to touch the tip of your nose with your eyes shut. But without gravity's pull on your limbs' stretch receptors, their proprioceptive data goes offline and arms and legs can go missing. An Apollo astronaut recounted his unsettling experience:

> The first night in space when I was drifting off to sleep, I
> suddenly realised that I had lost track of … my arms and legs.
> For all my mind could tell, my limbs were not there. However,
> with a conscious command for an arm or leg to move, it
> instantly reappeared – only to disappear again when I relaxed.[2]

Lacking up, down, and even at times apparently lacking limbs, space sickness is an unsettling experience. Thankfully, astronauts usually adapt to the disconcerting environment after a few days. One space traveller who certainly did not adapt was Utah Senator Jake Garn. In 1985 Garn, then 52, became the first sitting member of Congress to travel in space when he was invited aboard the *Discovery* shuttle. His role on the mission was to be a guinea pig for space sickness experiments. Immediately after launch on April 12, Garn began feeling ill. Experiments fell by the wayside as Garn became incapacitated by nausea and vomiting. When they finally landed eight days later Garn needed physical assistance just to get off the shuttle. Unsurprisingly, that journey was Garn's only space flight. Despite his brief career with NASA, his name lives on in the form of the Garn scale: an informal method of quantifying space sickness. NASA physician Robert Stevenson explained:

> ... Garn has made a mark in the Astronaut Corps because he represents the maximum level of space sickness that anyone can ever attain, and so the mark of being totally sick and totally incompetent is one Garn. Most guys will get maybe to a tenth Garn, if that high.[3]

In space, no one can hear you ask for a bucket.

*

Vomiting. Everything about it is repellent: its texture, its colour, its taste, its sound as it spatters into the toilet bowl. Perversely, for some people, vomit's only redeeming feature is its smell. Humans, being the impressionable creatures that we are, can be tricked into enjoying the smell of vomit if blindfolded and told that we're whiffing freshly grated Parmesan cheese. Butyric acid gives both chunky yellow substances their distinctive aroma.

But before we get to vomiting, we need to consider nausea: the feeling that you're about to spew. It can begin subtly as a lump at the back of your throat, or an awareness of your stomach. Some people describe a sensation of warmth and general malaise. You might burp, salivate or break into a sweat.

If you want to experience nausea, there are several things you could try. Skol some rancid milk. Have a general anaesthetic. Get pregnant. Listen to an Oscars acceptance speech. But perhaps the most reliable nausea trigger is motion, particularly low-frequency rocking like the undulating roll aboard a ship. Over 2000 years ago Hippocrates wrote that 'sailing on the sea proves that motion disorders the body'. Motion sickness is so intrinsic to seafaring that the association is embedded in the word 'nausea', which comes from the Ancient Greek *naus* meaning ship (the fact that nausea ends in '-sea' is just a happy coincidence).

A survey of more than 20,000 passengers from 114 sea voyages found that 21 per cent felt 'slightly unwell' while at sea, four per cent felt 'quite ill', another four per cent felt 'absolutely dreadful' and seven per cent vomited.[4] But a tendency to spew at sea need not preclude a stellar career in the navy: Admiral Horatio Nelson suffered debilitating seasickness. In 1804, a year before his Battle of Trafalgar victory, Nelson revealed in a letter: 'I am ill every time it blows hard and nothing but my enthusiastic love for my profession keeps me one hour at sea.'[5]

Most people will suffer motion sickness at some stage in their life. Women are more susceptible than men, and migraine sufferers are particularly prone. Children are resistant to motion sickness before the age of two, their sensitivity peaks around age nine, then things will usually settle down into adulthood.

Motion sickness happens when your brain receives conflicting messages about whether your body is moving or not. Two sources provide the brain with movement data: your eyes, and a section of your inner ear. You're probably vaguely aware that your inner ears have something to do with balance – indeed, your ears aren't just for hearing, they're responsible for keeping you upright.

The bit we're interested in is called your inner ear, but it's only about four centimetres (1.5 inches) in from your earhole. First comes the external ear: the bit you can get pierced, plus the waxy tube leading to your eardrum. Behind the eardrum is your middle ear, housing a chain of bones which transmit your eardrum's vibrations to the inner ear. And already, we've arrived at our destination. Here, in each inner ear, lie a pair of connected fluid-filled structures: your cochlea (for detecting sound), and what's called your vestibular system – the bit responsible for balance.

Your cochlea and vestibular system have quite a lot in common. Both inner ear structures rely on their internal fluid currents to interpret sound or balance data from your environment. For the cochlea, it's sound waves that generate the currents. For your vestibular system, it's both your head movements and gravity that shift the fluid. Both structures are lined with thousands of hair cells which sway to and fro in the currents – like seaweed in the shallows. Whenever a hair cell bends it generates a nerve signal that it sends to your brain. Your brain interprets bending hair cell data from your cochlea as sound, and infers your head position and whether you're upright based on your vestibular system's hair cell data.

Your inner ear resembles an avant garde sculpture in a modern art gallery. At the base is the cochlea, shaped like the shell of a snail. Your vestibular system extends from the cochlea where the snail's head would be. It begins as a bulbous knob called the 'vestibule' (from the Latin for 'entrance court', since it's like your cochlea's lobby). It ends with three looping tubes called the semicircular canals – specifically, the horizontal, posterior and superior canals, named after the direction of head movement they detect.

Without this knob-and-loop structure within each inner ear you'd lose track of your head's position and you'd struggle to remain upright. Here's why. The three semicircular canals keep track of your head's rotation. Your head can rotate in three planes – nodding (sensed by the superior canal), shaking your head like you're saying 'no' (horizontal canal), and flopping your head side to side against your shoulders (posterior canal). Nodding your head down, for example, sends a wave of fluid from the back of your head towards your nose inside each inner ear's superior semicircular canal. As the waves crash onto hair cells at the front of the canals, their bending generates a nerve signal that your brain interprets as: 'chin has been lowered towards chest'. By simultaneously combining the input from each inner ear's three canals, your brain can detect head rotation in any direction.

Your vestibular system's vestibule (that bulbous knob part, the 'lobby' to the cochlea) keeps track of where the ground and sky are by detecting changes in your head's position with respect to gravity. Hair cells within the vestibule are entombed in gloopy gel. The gel's surface is studded with a layer of calcium carbonate crystals called otoconia. Although otoconia literally means 'ear dust', these crystals are heavy. No matter what position your head is in, gravity will drag the heavy layer of crystals towards the ground, bending the hair cells with them. When you're upright, for example, the crystals evenly squash the hair cells beneath, telling your brain that 'down' is directly beneath your feet. If you're lying on your back in bed, gravity causes the crystal layer to sag towards your pillow, dragging the hair cells with it. Your brain can infer from the hair cells' position that now 'down' is under the back of your head.

As well as keeping tabs on up and down, the vestibule can also detect changes in linear acceleration. Imagine you're running late for work. You're stopped in your car at a red traffic light when, finally, it turns green. When you stomp on the accelerator your head is shoved backwards into the headrest because for a fraction of a second, your car is moving forward, but your body remains stationary. Within your vestibules, the same backward shearing force on the hair cells allows your brain to detect the acceleration.

With those principles in mind, we can finally explain why you feel nauseated in a boat or car, why astronauts feel topsy-turvy, and why the world won't stop spinning when you step off a playground roundabout.

Say you're reading this page as a passenger in a moving car. Your inner ears can detect that you're in motion: your vestibules sense the vehicle's acceleration and deceleration. But from your eyes' perspective, you're still. They are staring at this text framed by the stationary interior of the vehicle. You could be reading in a parked car for all your eyes know, but your inner ears say you're moving. Which message should your brain believe? Home videos with shaky camerawork can trigger motion sickness via the opposite sensory mismatch: your eyes tracking the rapid panning think you're moving, but reclined on the couch, your stagnant inner ear fluid tells your brain that you're still. Whichever way around the conflict is, your brain becomes bamboozled by the clashing information it is being fed. Are you moving, or not? This internal turmoil defines motion sickness.

When astronauts launch into space they leave behind their friends, their family, and a functional vestibular system. Humans, and our vestibular systems, evolved on a planet with gravity. To discern up from down, your vestibules rely on that gravity dragging their heavy gloop-entombed crystals towards the floor. Without gravity's familiar pull, the vestibules become defunct and the astronaut's brain is left in the lurch. Hence cosmonaut Titov's 'flying upside-down' experience.

Spinning rapidly in a circle sets up a current within the fluid in your semicircular canals. Say you're gleefully whirling around on your office chair when your boss unexpectedly enters the room. When you grab your desk, your body will stop moving, but the fluid whirling through the semicircular canals in your inner ears won't. You'll experience a nauseating visual illusion of the room rotating around you, called vertigo. You can speed up your recovery by spinning on your chair in the opposite direction. But your boss probably won't be too impressed.

Office chair capers are common causes of vertigo in younger people, but vertigo in older people is often caused by dislodged otoconia. The condition is abbreviated to 'BPPV', standing for benign (it won't kill you) paroxysmal (every so often) positional (triggered by certain head movements) vertigo (spew-inducing room spinning). Those calcium carbonate crystals in your vestibules need to remain embedded in your vestibule's gel. If any of them break free, they can work their way into one of the three semicircular canals. This is a disaster. Since it's impossible to rotate only half of your head, any head movements normally generate balanced fluid currents through both ears' semicircular canals. That balance disappears if one ear has loose heavy crystals messing with its canals' fluid dynamics. Your brain can't comprehend the mismatched signal: how could one side of your head be rotating differently from the other? You experience this as a debilitating bout of vertigo every time you move your head in a particular direction (depending on which semicircular canal contains the wayward crystals). Treatment involves physical head manoeuvres that waft the recalcitrant crystals back into the vestibule, rather like those handheld games where you have to tilt a steel ball through a maze.

*

Having discussed the causes of nausea ad nauseam, it's time for the main event: vomiting.

Two hours after an iffy street-food dinner, you start to feel nauseated. Saliva pools in your mouth, you start sweating and your wiser kebab-shunning companion notes that you've turned alabaster. You try parting your parched lips to vocalise your queasiness only to be overcome by involuntary retching. Your abs contract as you repeatedly gag and splutter without bringing anything up. Suddenly, with an overwhelming sensation of losing control, the contents of your stomach unceremoniously spew out onto the kerb. Having returned your street food to the street, you feel weak and exhausted but immensely improved.

Like completing a tax return or cleaning your gutters, vomiting is dreadful at the time but ultimately worth it. Vomiting rids your body of swallowed toxins and harmful chemicals before they have a chance to wreak havoc deep inside you. This mechanism makes sense when you spew after eating an off kebab, but what about vomiting on a rocking boat? You haven't swallowed anything dodgy, so why vomit? The truth is we don't really know, but one theory is that your brain thinks that you've been poisoned.[6]

Cruise ships and cars represent very modern methods of baffling your brain with conflicting sensory data. For most of human evolution, the only time your brain dealt with confusing inputs was after eating a poisonous plant. Ingested plant chemicals can induce bewildering visual and auditory hallucinations. Morning Glory seeds (*Ipomoea violacea*), for example, contain lysergic acid amide (LSA), which closely resembles LSD and has similar psychedelic properties. Eating other plants like monkshood (*Aconitum*) can cause bizarre skin sensations like numbness and tingling despite nothing having touched your skin. When you're experiencing motion sickness, your brain's only explanation for the conflicting inputs is that you've been poisoned. The appropriate response, then, is to vomit to remove the toxin from your system.

In the moments before you vomit your body makes some rapid protective adaptations. Stomach acid in spew can erode the enamel on your teeth. Pumping out extra saliva protects your teeth somewhat via a layer of viscous drool. Just before you vomit you reflexively take in a deep breath. This protects your lungs from becoming vomit-clogged by your attempts to breathe mid-evacuation.

Next comes the gut churning. Your small intestine starts squeezing backwards from about midway along its length. As its contents backtrack towards your stomach, your abdominal muscles squeeze tightly. This high pressure in your abdomen, plus low pressure in your chest (remember that big breath you took in) help force the vomit upwards. The ring of muscle at the base of your oesophagus – your lower oesophageal sphincter – loosens to prepare for the imminent eruption. Finally, your gut contents are propelled up, through your oesophagus and out of your mouth.

Vomiting clearly involves some complex choreography. The vomiting centre – despite sounding like an unappealing shopping destination – is the area of your brainstem that decides when you throw up. It bases its decision on inputs from multiple sources. Hair cell data from your vestibular system provides key intelligence. If your gastrointestinal tract distends, becomes blocked or has its lining irritated (by ingested microbes in kebab meat, or swallowed blood [see *Nosebleeds*, page 107], for example), it will liaise with your vomiting centre to initiate a spew. Brain networks involved with intense emotions like pain (like breaking a bone, or having a heart attack), disgust (such as seeing another person vomit), and fear (before a public-speaking engagement, for instance) influence the vomiting centre too.

The vomiting centre's final major informant is a small patch of the brain that's particularly sensitive to chemicals, hence its name: the chemoreceptor trigger zone (CTZ). Sitting conveniently just beside your vomiting centre, the CTZ has serious sway over the vomiting centre's decisions. General anaesthetic drugs and chemotherapy are particularly strong CTZ irritants. As is human chorionic gonadotropin (hCG), the hormone produced by a developing placenta that makes that second blue line appear on a urine pregnancy test. Since two placentas pump out more hCG than one, women expecting twins can experience worse nausea and vomiting than those incubating a singleton. Morning-sickness is a misnomer – the nausea can occur at any time of day. Thankfully, by about 14 weeks placental hCG production starts to fall and the nausea usually subsides.

Because vomiting is such an unpleasant experience, we tend to avoid situations that previously caused us to vomit. Psychologists call this conditioning. For example, if you suffered food poisoning after eating a prawn, you'll probably be turned off prawns for life. Just looking at a prawn could make you feel queasy. The same phenomenon can occur in patients receiving multiple doses of chemotherapy. If an early dose makes them intensely unwell, their brain becomes conditioned to associate chemotherapy with vomiting. Thinking about chemotherapy, driving into the hospital carpark or hearing the beep of an IV pump can trigger a vomit. I cared for a patient who retched at the smell of alcohol swabs: a conditioned response from chemotherapy he'd received decades earlier when being treated for lung cancer. Up to 25 per cent of patients receiving chemotherapy suffer from this anticipatory nausea and vomiting by the time they reach their fourth chemotherapy dose.[7] Some patients find it so distressing that they stop taking chemotherapy altogether. Prevention is the best treatment: taking strong anti-nausea medications right from the start of treatment stops the brain from making the negative nausea associations.

The high pressures involved in vomiting can tear your oesophagus along its length. Without surgery, this condition is universally fatal. Oesophageal rupture is known as Boerhaave syndrome, after Dutch physician Herman Boerhaave who published a blow-by-blow description of the process in 1723.[8] The victim was Baron Jan van Wassenaer, 'a man of fifty years, and of powerful frame' who was known as a 'gross feeder'. Boerhaave wrote: 'At the time of the accident which caused his death, Baron de Wassenaer was atoning by low diet for an excess at table committed three days before.' The Baron's 'low diet' sounded quite generous:

Veal soup, with herbs; boiled lamb and cabbage; fried sweetbread and spinach; duck; two larks; compote of apples; dessert, pears, grapes, sweetmeats; beer and moselle.

Following this heavy meal, the Baron:

… began to complain of the old disagreeable feeling about the stomach, and he swallowed three tumblerfuls of a hot infusion of thistle. As this did not act with its usual efficacy, he took four more glasses of the same infusion, but still without effect. Much surprised at this, the Baron ordered another dose to be prepared, and in the meantime strove to excite vomiting by tickling his [tonsils]. Whilst straining violently he suddenly felt a horrible pain and gave such a cry of anguish that his servants hastened to his assistance. He exclaimed that something had burst or been violently displaced near the pit of his stomach, and that he was sure he must die immediately.

He was right. The Baron's vigorous vomiting had torn his oesophagus down its length, providing a swift and permanent end to his dietary woes.

SUMMARY: Motion sickness makes you feel nauseated because your brain doesn't know if you're moving or not. Chemicals, gut disturbances and strong emotions can make you nauseated too. Nausea can culminate in vomiting, your body's way of removing harmful ingested toxins.

AND ALSO ...

The (very few) benefits of vomiting

Tactical vomiting is the practice of self-inflicted vomiting during an alcohol binge, performed to feel well enough to continue the festivities. Contrary to popular myth, the vomitorium of an ancient Roman venue was not the area where Romans engaged in tactical vomiting to make room for more feasting. Instead, the vomitorium was the series of passageways through which the crowd exited (literally, spewed out) from the main seating area.

Other species besides *Homo sapiens* engage in tactical vomiting. Killer whales have been observed using their vomit as bait. The whale will surreptitiously surface, spew, then retreat to loiter just below the waves until a hungry gull hits the water. As the gullible gull tucks into the bobbing orca vomit, the whale will surge, mouth open, and swallow the gull whole.

Vultures tactically vomit when cornered by a predator. Vomiting has two advantages for the vulture. Firstly, it makes the bird lighter, enabling it to fly away more easily. Secondly, it provides a decoy for the predator, who may choose to eat the vomit rather than waste energy pursuing the vulture. You've got to admire the cold hard logic of that decision.

Neigh, a horse can't vomit

Rodents – gnawing mammals like squirrels and rats – can't vomit. This is why rat poison works so well; once the poison is down, the rat can't rectify its error with a healthy chuck. Horses can't vomit either. Horses have an incredibly strong ring of muscle where the oesophagus meets the stomach, called the lower oesophageal sphincter. The sphincter is so strong that it's physically unable to relax to permit vomiting. This digestive system quirk may have evolved to help horses flee predators. At full gallop, a horse's intestines repeatedly slam into its stomach like a piston. If the same stomach hammering happened inside us, the pressure would pop open our weakling lower oesophageal sphincter immediately, shooting our breakfast all over the floor. But a horse's iron-clad lower oesophageal sphincter allows them to hold on to both their lunch and their life as they gallop to safety. Although horses might be able to escape wolves, wolfing down contaminated food could kill them instead.

Gag me with a spoon

The gag reflex is a sudden throat contraction triggered by anything touching the back of your tongue, throat or around your tonsils. You might have experienced this during overzealous teeth brushing, or when a doctor clumsily squashed your tongue to peer at your tonsils. The gag reflex protects you from choking: anything big enough to scrape the top of your throat probably won't fit down your oesophagus. Before you choke, the gagging ejects the culprit straight back out. If your gag reflex is too strong however, you might end up vomiting. Testing a patient's gag reflex is part of a thorough medical examination, since an absent reflex can indicate neurological disease. At medical school, the importance of standing to one side during this examination is emphasised, lest the patient vomit in your face.

Doing the Bush thing

Midway through a tour of Asia in January 1992, President George H. W. Bush was enjoying a banquet held by the Japanese Prime Minister Kiichi Miyazawa. Bush had just tucked into the second course of caviar with raw salmon. Before the third course arrived (pepper sauce over grilled beef) he began feeling nauseated. Suddenly, in front of 135 diplomats, Bush vomited all over the Prime Minister's pants, then fainted in his lap. Upon regaining consciousness and becoming aware of his mortifying conduct Bush moaned: 'roll me under the table until the dinner's over'. The infamous event, later attributed to food poisoning, gave rise to a Japanese euphemism for vomiting: *bushusuru*, literally meaning 'to do the Bush thing'.

A not-so-healthy glow

Matchmaking was a big industry in Britain in the 1850s (I mean literally making matches, not setting up single people on dates). Victorian homes were lit by candles and gas lamps which required a ready source of flame. Women working in matchstick factories suffered terribly from the toxic effects of white phosphorus, a component of the match heads. The women nicknamed the syndrome 'phossy jaw'. It started with a toothache and swollen gums before the entire lower jaw decayed. Since phosphorus is fluorescent, the rotting jawbone glowed green in the dark. Swallowed phosphorus caused vomiting, and the vomit also glowed:

> The grandchildren of East Enders who lived near the factory recall tales of their glowing piles of fluorescent vomit which marked the ... workers' homeward routes at the end of each shift.[9]

ENDNOTES

1   Golightly, G. Flying The Vomit Comet Has Its Ups And Downs. *Space.com* (20 October 1999). https://web.archive.org/web/20060310204522/http://www. space.com/peopleinterviews/yaniec_991020.html.

2   Clément, G. & Reschke, M. F. *Neuroscience in Space.* Springer Science & Business Media (2010).

3   Evans, B. *Tragedy and triumph in orbit: the Eighties and early Nineties.* Springer (2012)

4   Lawther A. & Griffin M. J. A survey of the occurrence of motion sickness amongst passengers at sea. *Aviation Space Environmental Medicine*, 59, 399 (1988).

5   Brown, K. *The seasick admiral: Nelson and the health of the Navy.* Seaforth Publishing (2015).

6   Treisman, M. Motion sickness: an evolutionary hypothesis. *Science Magazine*, 197 (4302), 493–495 (1977).

7   Aapro, M. S. et al. Anticipatory nausea and vomiting. *Supportive Care in Cancer*, 13 (2), 117–121 (2004).

8   Barrett, N. R. Spontaneous Perforation of the Oesophagus: Review of the Literature and Report of Three New Cases. *Thorax*, 1 (1), 48–70 (1946).

9   Raw, L. *Striking a light: the Bryant and May Matchwomen and their place in history.* Continuum (2011).

DIARRHOEA
Hard to spell and equally hard to endure.

Bristol, in England's south-west corner, is known for its suspension bridge and 'irrepressible creative spirit', according to its gushing tourism website. But in medical circles, the city is also known for its stool chart. When I was an intern working on a gastroenterology ward, the Bristol Stool Chart, a seven-point scale to describe the consistency of human faeces, was provided to me as a laminated card. Type 1 is 'separate hard lumps'; type 4 is the Goldilocks 'smooth soft sausage or snake'; type 7 is 'liquid consistency with no solid pieces' – diarrhoea. For the ward's Christmas party, a nurse baked a cake topped with a confectionary representation of each stool type. Starting from type 1, the cake was a spectacular display of the Chart: choc-chips, a Picnic bar, a Flake, a Mars bar, dobs of praline, a streak of chocolate buttercream, and a pool of chocolate syrup.

Rather than rely on chocolate bars, toilet bowl and cistern manufacturers have created a real recipe to replicate faeces: a mix of soybean paste with rice, extruded into 50-gram (1.7 ounce) cylinders using a sausage maker. These standardised fake stools are needed to assess the cistern's flush mechanisms. The soybean-based recipe was found, after extensive testing, to best mirror human faeces' moisture content, density, and propensity to break apart when flushed. Toilets are judged according to how many 50-gram cylinders they can clear with one flush. A bottom-of-the-range loo must be able to flush five soy cylinders (250 grams/8.8 ounces) in a single flush (250 grams being the average man's maximal faecal mass as determined by a landmark 1978 study 'Variability of colonic function in healthy subjects' published in the self-explanatorily titled journal *Gut*).[1]

To earn a 'high-efficiency' label, the US Environmental Protection Agency requires the toilet to clear seven soy cylinders (350 grams/12 ounces) of waste in one flush using no more than 4.8 litres (10 pints) of water. Top-notch loos can flush a hefty 20 soy cylinders (one kilogram/35 ounces). It's unclear why such a powerful flush capacity is necessary, unless you're a man who only flushes after every fourth defecation.

*

The food you eat takes a long and winding route through your guts before it emerges from your anus as a 50-gram (1.7 ounce), soybean-paste-like cylinder. If things go wrong along that journey – through your small, then large intestine – diarrhoea can result.

The small intestine is 'small' in the same way Turkish delight is 'delightful': it's not. It's actually six metres (about 20 feet) long with a surface area equivalent to two car parking spaces. The 'small' refers to its three-centimetre (about one-inch) calibre, compared to the wider six-centimetre (2.3 inch) 'large' bowel. (On semantics: 'bowel' covers the entirety of the small and large intestine, but 'colon' applies only to the large intestine.) Intestines, small or large, are muscular tubes with an absorbent lining. Their job is to suck out the nutrients from everything you swallow, propelling the dregs along and absorbing water until a 250-gram (8.8-ounce) Bristol Stool Chart type 4 specimen is ready for evacuation.

The time it takes for a bite of food to pass between your facial cheeks and your buttock cheeks varies wildly. The stomach takes two to five hours to empty. Another two to six hours elapse before the small intestine squeezes out its contents. Finally, the large intestine enjoys a leisurely 10 to 60 hours of stool contact before final evacuation. This prolonged exposure to potential carcinogens in your food is one reason why large intestine cancers are so much more common than small intestinal ones. A normal range for total gut transit is anything from 24 to 72 hours.

Jet-setting human drug mules can exploit their gut transit time to transport swallowed contraband-packed condoms. This is an incredibly dangerous pursuit. Usually, the worst-case scenario of condom rupture is an unplanned pregnancy, but here the stakes are even higher: if the condom splits in the trafficker's intestines, the ensuing massive overdose of cocaine or heroin is usually lethal. Successful 'body packers' must keep these wads of drugs intact and hidden in their intestines until they land and find a private privy to evacuate their valuable cargo. Efforts to slow their gut transit time are necessary if their journey involves stop-overs between long-haul flights. Taking anti-diarrhoeal medication before take-off is a given. During the flight they won't eat or drink, since stomach filling hormonally triggers the intestines to start squeezing. The cabin crew are trained to alert security if they identify a nervous passenger who refuses all meals.

Your small intestine has such a ludicrously large surface area because its walls are lined with finger-like projections called villi. You've got 10 to 40 villi per square millimetre of small intestine. These densely packed extensions, each 0.5 to 1 millimetre long, give your intestinal wall a luxurious, velvety appearance. Each villus is in turn covered in its own microscopic villi, adding even more surface area. To be absorbed, nutrients in your food must physically touch your small intestine's lining. A greater surface area means a greater chance that all the chemical nutrients in your food will be absorbed. After six metres (about 20 feet) of sucking up, a watery slurry of indigestible filler material – like plant fibres, sloughed off dead intestinal wall cells, and corn kernels – remains, ready to splash into the large intestine.

The transition point from your small to your large intestine is at the lower right-hand corner of your abdomen. If you've had your appendix out, this is where the scar will be: your appendix dangles off your large intestine just after the small-to-large intestine juncture. Your large intestine heads due north until your lower ribs, takes a 90-degree turn to cross to the left side of your body, then makes another 90-degree turn, heading due south to the lower left-hand corner of your abdomen. Your small intestine sits as a tangled mess in the centre of this 1.5-metre-long (five-foot-long) large intestinal frame. Stools back up at the end of your large intestine if you're constipated. A doctor can confirm that a left-sided lower abdominal mass is stool rather than some other lumpy organ because, as my anatomy textbook memorably taught me, 'one can form indents in a faecal mass via palpation through the abdominal wall'.

Your large intestine's primary responsibility is to absorb water from the small intestine's dregs until a solid stool is formed. Normally your large intestine absorbs 99 per cent of the water you consume. And by 'water' I mean any liquid including coffee, milk, beer and wine (after all, once the dissolved sugar, colourings, alcohol and caffeine are absorbed, it's just water that's left). Let's imagine that you have been forced to drink 1.5 litres (three pints) of sarsaparilla (I assume nobody would voluntarily drink it) – only one tablespoon of sarsaparilla 'water' will end up in your faeces. Your large intestine will absorb the rest directly into your bloodstream. Cells in various organs will suck up whatever water they need as blood flows past them, then your kidneys will eliminate any excess water as urine. Diarrhoea happens if your large intestine fails to absorb the usual 99 per cent of water from your faeces.

The word diarrhoea literally means 'through flow' – from the Greek *dia* (through) and *rhoia* (flow). Three main problems result in through flow: undigested food making its way to your large intestine, damage to your intestinal lining, and acceleration of your intestinal squeezing rate.

Undigested food

Undigested food in your large intestine sucks in water via a process called osmosis. (Remember, all digestion should be complete once food hits your large intestine: it's just the water absorption that's left.) The extra water load overwhelms your large intestine's reabsorption abilities, resulting in diarrhoea. But why would undigested food make it to your large intestine? Well, either it wasn't digestible in the first place, or something went wrong upstream in the small intestine.

Consider the indigestible stuff first. Humans simply can't break down certain carbohydrates in plant foods referred to as fibre. Long ago in human evolution we forfeited the laborious ability to extract calories from grass when we developed the skills to cook nutrient-dense meat (see *Farts and burps*, page 212). Artificial sugar substitutes like saccharin are completely indigestible: after satisfying your sweet tooth, these chemicals travel through your guts without any nutrient (i.e. calorie) absorption.

In 1996, *The Lancet* published the mysteriously titled case study: 'An air stewardess with puzzling diarrhoea'.[2] This otherwise healthy 32-year-old woman was having up to ten loose stools a day. Against all the odds the culprit was not dodgy airline food, but her habit of constantly chewing 'sugar-free' gum, which is loaded with the indigestible sugar sorbitol. You need to chew enormous quantities of sorbitol-sweetened gum before diarrhoea results: our luckless stewardess was getting through 75 grams (2.6 ounces) of sorbitol a day (a stick of sugar-free gum has about 1.25 grams). Presumably, because her job required fresh breath, her daily quota of 60 sticks of gum and subsequent hospital admission with diarrhoea were tax-deductible.

Other foods, particularly sugars in fruits and dairy, *are* digestible – but only in small quantities. Lactose is the main sugar in breastmilk (and all milk, for that matter). Humans are born with the ability to make lactase, the digestive enzyme that breaks down lactose. Since breastmilk is usually a baby's sole source of nutrition for at least the first six months of its life, this is obviously a crucial enzyme to possess. Up until about 20,000 years ago, most humans lost the ability to produce lactase as they grew up. This made sense at a time when breastmilk was the only milk humans drank: why waste energy as an adult making the enzyme required to digest a food that only babies ate?

This all changed when Northern Europeans embraced cow's milk as a year-round source of handy nutrition. A genetic mutation in the population meant that some of these Europeans retained their lactase-making ability forever, not just in infancy. When crops failed, these mutants' lactase enzymes allowed them to survive the famine by drinking cow's milk. Any adults without the mutation – those who didn't make lactase – couldn't digest the lactose in the cow's milk, which passed straight through them and caused profuse diarrhoea (as anyone with lactose intolerance today will understand). Without the cow's milk for nutrition, people who couldn't digest lactose were more likely to starve.

In warmer equatorial destinations like Asia and Africa, non-human milk never gained much traction as a reliable source of nutrition. Unrefrigerated dairy, sitting out in the Saharan sun, doesn't remain edible for long. As such, the 'make lactase forever' genetic mutation never took hold in these areas because it didn't offer any survival advantage. Modern rates of lactose intolerance reflect these global differences in reliance on milk for nutrition. A 2017 study published in *The Lancet* found very low rates of lactose intolerance among Danish (4 per cent), Swedish (7 per cent) and Dutch (12 per cent) citizens, compared to sky-high rates of intolerance in Japan (73 per cent), China (85 per cent) and Ghana (100 per cent).[3] But even the Dutch might have to lay off the Edam for a while after a gut infection. Lactase is produced in the tips of your small intestinal villi. If these are damaged by a bout of gastro, you might find that you're temporarily lactose-intolerant.

Even if a food *is* digestible, it may not be digested if things go wrong upstream of the large intestine. Food entering the small intestine is met with a stream of bile from the gallbladder and a squirt of juice from the pancreas. Each organ's secretions contain digestive enzymes that accelerate nutrient breakdown. Bile is also an emulsifier: it helps the fat in your food dissolve in those enzyme-rich watery secretions, rather than just float on their surface. A diseased gallbladder (blocked by a stone, for example) or pancreas (like one scarred from chronic alcohol use, or previous infection) can't secrete its enzyme-rich juices, allowing food to pass along undigested to your large intestine. Antibiotics might kill the bacteria responsible for your middle ear infection, but they also obliterate the friendly gut bacteria that help break down your food. This collateral damage means fewer bacteria remain to keep up with the usual level of food breakdown.

Like all organs, your guts need a blood supply to work. Diversion of blood flow away from the small intestine impairs food absorption, allowing undigested remnants to flow straight into your large intestine. Intense stress is a particularly effective way to deprive your intestines of blood. Adrenaline is a stress hormone that reroutes blood away from your guts towards your lungs (to pick up oxygen) and muscles (to deliver that oxygen, allowing you to flee or fight the source of stress). When your life is in danger, digestion can wait; self-preservation comes first. Adrenaline's blood-shunting effects – plus its ability to hasten intestinal squeezing, as we will soon discover – explains why many athletes, public speakers and exam candidates suffer the additional stress of a dose of diarrhoea before their big event.

A damaged intestinal lining

Now that we've digested the problems with undigested food, let's consider the second major diarrhoea culprit: a damaged intestinal lining. Diarrhoea due to intestinal infection from contaminated food is called gastroenteritis or food poisoning. Gastro-causing pathogens invade and rupture the cells that make up your intestinal lining. Burst villi in your small intestine can't absorb nutrients (causing diarrhoea via the 'undigested food' mechanism again) while an obliterated large intestinal lining can't absorb water. Bacteria like *Salmonella*, *E. coli* and *Campylobacter* work in this way, as do viruses like rotaviruses – typically responsible for outbreaks of kindergarten gastro – and noroviruses – the classic cause of gastro aboard cruise ships.

Inflammatory bowel disease refers to two conditions – ulcerative colitis (UC) and Crohn's disease – in which a rogue immune system causes constant intestinal inflammation. The red, swollen lining can't function, resulting in diarrhoea.

In UC, which spares the small intestine, gradual erosion of the large intestine's lining severely affects its water-absorbing abilities. As expected, diarrhoea can be copious in UC. Gastroenterologists use a standardised scale to classify how severe a patient's UC flare is. Diarrhoea up to three times a day is considered a 'mild' flare; the 'severe' label is reserved for those who suffer at least six bouts of diarrhoea per day, with visible blood. Incidentally, UC is one of the only medical conditions (another being Parkinson's disease) where smoking is protective. Smokers are less likely to develop UC in the first place, people with UC who smoke have less severe flares than non-smokers, and if a person with UC takes up smoking, they often experience marked clinical improvement. But the litany of health risks associated with smoking, including shaving a decade off your life expectancy, definitely outweigh any benefits.

Crohn's disease, the other inflammatory bowel disease, tends to affect women (which is unfortunate given the homophone 'crone' means 'an ugly hag'). Unlike UC, which only involves the large intestine, Crohn's disease causes inflammation throughout the small intestine too, resulting in a double-whammy diarrhoea mechanism via impaired upstream digestion too.

An accelerated intestinal squeezing rate

The third and final diarrhoea mechanism is pretty self-evident: if your intestines squeeze too quickly there won't be enough time for adequate nutrient and water absorption. Moving food through your intestines relies on peristalsis: sequential muscular contractions along the intestines which propel your soon-to-be-stool in the desired direction. Once or twice a day your large intestine undergoes a 'mass movement' or 'giant migrating contraction' (those are legitimate medical terms, I swear). Usually triggered by eating (your intestines need to make room for the food hitting your stomach), long segments of your large intestine vigorously contract and completely empty. If you routinely defecate every morning after breakfast, your mass movement into the toilet bowl was likely the result of a mass movement in your large intestine.

Between heroic mass movements, smaller-scale gentle peristalsis keeps your intestinal contents shuffling along. Just like your heart pumps at a regular rate, so too do your intestines. A dense network of nerves laces your intestinal walls. When one of these nerves fires, the surrounding portion of intestinal muscle squeezes and the stool inside is pushed along. The nerve firing rate is determined by pacemaker cells called the 'interstitial cells of Cajal' which discharge like clockwork at a regular frequency: every 7 seconds in your small intestine and every 20 seconds in your large intestine. The exotic name is a nod to their discoverer Santiago Ramón y Cajal (1852-1934), a fiery Spanish neuroanatomist who, at the age of 11, built a cannon and exploded his neighbour's side gate. Similarly explosive diarrhoea can result from anything that excites Cajal's cells.

These cells are exquisitely sensitive to chemicals including adrenaline, ethanol, caffeine, and laxatives like senna and castor oil. Castor oil was used to lubricate the rotary engines of planes during World War I. After a few hours flying, the pilots' bowels reliably turned to water due to the effects of the ingested aerosolised castor oil fumes. The extra adrenaline from the stress of being shot at by the enemy probably exacerbated matters too.

A 1949 experiment on unsuspecting medical students elegantly demonstrated adrenaline's role in increasing intestinal contractions.[4] The students agreed to undergo a colonoscopy, under the pretence of being healthy control subjects for some later trial. A researcher would casually chat with the student while inserting a colonoscope – with a concealed pressure gauge – into the student's rectum. Suddenly the researcher would stop talking, as though something had gone wrong. He would call in a colleague and announce in a stage whisper that he had identified what looked to be a rectal cancer. Lo and behold, the student's rate of large intestinal contractions, measured by the secret pressure gauge, went through the roof. At this point the hoax was revealed, and the contractions immediately abated. Apparently, the students all found this hilarious and none of them complained that their rights had been violated. Ah, the 1940s.

SUMMARY: Diarrhoea is the result of too much water in your faeces. Achieving that elusive Bristol Stool Chart type 4 stool requires everything you eat to be fully digested, an intact intestinal lining, and a steady intestinal squeezing rate.

AND ALSO …

Don't drink from the Broad Street well

Vibrio cholerae, the bacteria responsible for cholera, causes diarrhoea via an ingenious mechanism: it produces a toxin that dupes the large intestine into pumping water into the stool rather than sucking it out. The result is voluminous so-called 'rice water' diarrhoea. Dehydration is profound in cholera and can kill within hours if untreated. Hospitals in endemic areas are furnished with cholera cots: specially designed beds with a hole in the middle for the patient's backside. The patient lies on the bed, buttocks positioned over the hole, with a bucket underneath to catch the near-constant diarrhoeal flow.

There have been seven cholera pandemics in the past 200 years, the first originating in India in 1817. When the third pandemic hit London in 1853, *The Lancet*'s editor Thomas Wakely lamented:

> ... all is darkness and confusion, vague theory, and a vain speculation. Is it a fungus, an insect, a miasma, an electrical disturbance, a deficiency of ozone, a morbid off-scouring from the intestinal canal? We know nothing; we are at sea in a whirlpool of conjecture.[5]

London physician John Snow took a rather less melodramatic approach, reasoning that:

> The morbid material producing cholera must be introduced into the alimentary canal – must, in fact, be swallowed accidentally, for persons would not take it intentionally.[6]

Soho, in London's West End, suffered a particularly severe cholera outbreak in 1854. In the 10 days between 31 August and 10 September some 500 people died. Snow meticulously plotted every case on a map of Soho, trying to determine the source of the 'morbid material'. Snow's investigation revealed that:

> ... there had been no particular outbreak or increase of cholera in this part of London, except among the persons who were in the habit of drinking the water from the [Broad Street] pipe-well.

Snow convinced London officials to dismantle the pump's handle, making it impossible to draw water from the well. Cholera cases immediately plummeted. It turns out the well had been dug right next to a leaky cesspit teeming with *Vibrio cholerae.*

Soft stools, hard bug

Marjorie was a memorable octogenarian I looked after when I was working as a general medical registrar. She had a gut infection due to a bacterium called *Clostridium difficile.* The *difficile* refers to its obstinate refusal to grow in petri dishes. But it's a *difficile* bug to treat too. Marjorie experienced a dreaded complication called 'toxic megacolon', which is exactly what it sounds like: her large intestine swelled up to enormous proportions and almost burst. After two months in hospital receiving heavy-duty antibiotics to kill the *Clostridium difficile* in her gut, her intractable diarrhoea finally began to ease. One day I was with another patient when I heard her shriek my name: 'Sarah! Quick!' I sprinted down the corridor, expecting to find her sprawled on the ground with a broken hip. Instead, she was pointing at the toilet bowl with tears in her eyes. Puzzled, I peered in. There was a smooth, soft sausage. 'I'm back to type fours!' Overjoyed, we hugged each other. After she'd washed her hands.

ENDNOTES

1 Wyman, J. B. et al. Variability of colonic function in healthy subjects. *Gut*, 19 (2), 146–150 (1978).

2 Greaves, R. et al. An air stewardess with puzzling diarrhoea. *The Lancet*, 348 (9040), 1488 (1996).

3 Storhaug, C. et al. Country, regional, and global estimates for lactose malabsorption in adults: a systematic review and meta-analysis. *The Lancet Gastroenterology & Hepatology*, 2 (10), 738–746 (2017).

4 Almy, T et al. Alterations in Colonic Function in Man Under Stress. *Gastroenterology*, 12 (3), 425–436 (1949).

5 Wakley, T. *The Lancet II*, p. 393 (1853).

6 Snow, J. *On the Mode of Communication of Cholera.* John Churchill, New Burlington Street, England (1855).

FARTS AND BURPS

Death, taxes and making gas. These are life's certainties.

The bizarre ending to the 1956 Aintree Grand National steeplechase has never been explained. Devon Loch, the Queen Mother's thoroughbred, was coasting to victory when the 10-year-old gelding inexplicably collapsed 50 metres (164 feet) from the finish line. 'He's slipped! He's down!' cried the horrified commentator. But Devon Loch didn't simply slip. The horse's body abruptly launched into the air before he bellyflopped on the turf with all four legs splayed. Hopes of a royal victory vanished as the other runners sailed past him.

Theories ran riot in the racing community. Some said Devon Loch had jumped an imaginary fence. Others suggested he'd been spooked by the raucous crowd. But another explanation was less savoury: *The Guardian* reported that Devon Loch had become 'destabilised by breaking wind violently after his girth was made too tight'.[1] After galloping nearly seven kilometres (over four miles) and jumping over 30 fences with a vice-like girth around his belly, the poor horse emitted such a violent fart that it propelled him into the air like a rocket. The combined embarrassment of farting in public, falling over, and losing a race must have left Devon Loch mortified. Particularly since he knew that the Queen and her mum were watching.

Fart control in other animals is far superior to that in horses. Manatees, also known as sea cows, rely on farting to control their buoyancy. Releasing a fart allows the manatee to sink deeper below the water. If a manatee becomes constipated, its inability to fart leaves it bobbing helplessly on the water's surface with its tail above its head. Birds and sloths are perhaps the masters of fart control: they don't fart at all. Northern Europeans take fart control particularly seriously. Or should I say *fartkontrol*. Fart means 'fast' in several Scandinavian languages. In Denmark, an area of road where speed is being monitored is dubbed a *fartkontrol*. Signs next to speed bumps in Sweden read *farthinder*. It is with this juvenile mindset that we shall delve into the world of bodily gases.

*

Gases make a noise when they escape from your gastrointestinal tract. An oral escape is called a burp, belch or 'eructation', if you're a euphemistic doctor. An anal escape is a fart, flatus or flatulence. Gases within your intestinal tract can be noisy too. Empty stomachs can rumble as they knead air, as can segments of your intestine upon squeezing pockets of gas. Next time your innards start emitting these awkward sounds, consider muffling the gurgles by loudly telling your companions that their onomatopoeic medical name is 'borborygmus' (pronounced boar-boar-RIG-muss).

What would you estimate a human's average 24-hour fart volume to be? If you wanted to be scientific about it, you could poke a plastic tube up your rectum for a day, attach it to a bag and measure the volume of gas you'd collected the next morning. As it happens, this is precisely what ten volunteers submitted to in 1991. In the name of science, five men and five women aged between 19 and 25 agreed to the insertion of a 65-centimeter-long (two-foot-long) rectal tube to gather a day's worth of gas. They were required to consume a 200-gram (seven-ounce) can of baked beans (HP brand, in tomato sauce, supplied by the researchers), but the remainder of their diet was up to them. The results, published in the journal *Gut*, revealed that daily fart volume varied wildly from

467 to 1491 millilitres (about one to three pints), with an average of 705 millilitres (1.5 pints). Women and men produced similar amounts (in fact it was a woman who produced the largest volume). An average 'emission' averaged 90 millilitres (three fl oz). Peak gas production occurred during the day (averaging 34 millilitres /1.2 fl oz per hour), particularly following meals, then halved overnight (16 millilitres/0.5 fl oz per hour).

Six of the volunteers agreed to a second round with the tube, this time dining on fibre-free liquid meal supplements for 48 hours prior to and during the experiment. No other food was permitted besides black tea (presumably this was considered a basic human right by the research ethics committee; the study was performed in Sheffield, England, after all). On this diet, the average daily fart volume plummeted to just a third of the volume produced eating the beans-plus-whatever diet. The average daily fart number also dropped from nine to just 1.5.

What can we learn from this experiment, besides the fact that young people will volunteer for anything if they get free food? Everyone farts, your emissions could probably fill two beer cans per day, and fibre is to blame for a lot of that volume.

*

You've always got about 200 millilitres (7 fl oz) of gas within your gastrointestinal tract. That's assuming you're at sea level; at higher altitudes the lower air pressure will cause gases within you to expand. The propensity to fart on airplanes isn't just bad manners, it's physics. As the plane's height increases so does the volume of gas in your large intestine that's waiting to be released as a fart.

Let's take a brief mental tour through your gastrointestinal tract – from lips to anus – to see where these gases hide out.

Upon swallowing, your oesophagus squeezes your mouthful of baked beans into your stomach. Your stomach sloshes the beans around in hydrochloric acid for a few hours before releasing the mush into your small intestine. The mush is met with a wave of alkaline juices from your pancreas and gallbladder which rapidly neutralise the acid to prevent holes being burnt into your guts. Fat-dissolving emulsifiers and digestive enzymes in the fluid also start doing their jobs. Next comes the tedious six-metre (about 20-foot) journey along your small intestine during which nutrient extraction – digestion – takes place. The 'small' refers to the skinny width of the tube, not it's remarkable length. Eventually the nutrient-depleted dregs splash into your large intestine, whose mission is to suck water out of this slop and turn it into a solid stool by the time it has traversed its 1.5 metre (five foot) length. If all goes to plan, firm stool gradually accumulates in your rectum, the name assigned to the end of your large intestine. Stretch-sensitive nerves in your expanding rectum's walls fire off a message to your brain suggesting that you expel the growing faecal mass through a four-centimetre-long (1.5-inch-long) pipe called the anal canal, out of your anus, and into a lavatory (ideally).

Keeping faeces within your rectum until an appropriate private moment is an important social skill. Your anal anatomy ensures that unintentional spills are rare. Throughout your body, rings of muscles called sphincters control the flow of fluid through tubes. For instance, your lower oesophageal sphincter squeezes the end of your oesophagus shut between swallows to prevent stomach acid sloshing up your throat. Another sphincter orchestrates the flow from your stomach into your small intestine. Your sphincter of Oddi, nestled in the wall at the start of your small intestine, tightens and relaxes to control the addition of those alkaline juices to your incoming stomach contents.

Usually one sphincter does the job. But your anal canal is encircled by two strong sphincters to maintain faecal continence. If any bodily opening was going to have a back-up sphincter, you'd want it to be your anus. You've got no voluntary control over your internal anal sphincter, which is automatically clasped tight most of the time to stop fluid and farts indiscriminately leaking out of you. But your external anal sphincter, wrapped around the internal one, *is* under your control. Try to squeeze as though holding in a fart: you're activating your external anal sphincter.

Gas makes its way into your gastrointestinal tract in three ways. You can swallow it, it can pass through the gut wall from your blood, or it can form within the tract itself. Since your gastrointestinal tract only has two openings with the outside world, if the gas wants to escape your body it only has two choices: via your mouth (as a burp) or via your anus (as a fart). Let's start at the top.

Virtually all burping is due to swallowed air. Every normal swallow of saliva contains a few millilitres of air. Gulping down a meal is a particularly efficient way of aerating your stomach; each bite of a hamburger includes a bite of air too. Drinking carbonated drinks delivers gas directly into your stomach, which is why soft drinks (so-called because they lack 'hard' liquor) or carbonated hard drinks like beer are particularly burp-inducing. Chewing gum and smoking cigarettes can suck in extra air too.

As your stomach puffs up with gas, stretch-sensitive nerves in its walls (like the ones in your rectum) tell your lower oesophageal sphincter to momentarily relax. Suddenly, a northward escape route for gas trapped in your stomach appears. As the high-pressure gas whooshes up your oesophagus it sets the floppy tissues at the back of your throat vibrating, resulting in the characteristic sound of a burp. Forcing a burp out will make it louder. Just like inhaled helium can produce a squeaky voice, swallowed helium can produce squeaky burps. Some talented people, usually young men, learn to adjust the shape of their mouth and tongue to turn their burp-induced throat vibrations into 'burped speech'. Transforming throat vibrations into speech isn't just a juvenile party trick; it offers an alternate way of talking for people who have had their voice box surgically removed (usually due to cancer). Without vocal cords to act as noise generators, patients rely on throat vibrations to make a sound, which they learn to shape into words (see *Voice (loss of)*, page 147). An electronic device held to the throat is the conventional source of vibration, but burping would do the trick if the battery ran out.

Most swallowed air is burped straight back out, but posture has some influence on its chances of progressing through your gastrointestinal tract. Gas, being less dense than liquid, will always sit above any watery stomach contents. If you're sitting up, stomach gas will collect just below where the oesophagus joins your stomach, ready to be burped out. Stomach juices and food fills the rest of your stomach, plugged at the bottom by the sphincter leading to your small intestine. But if you stand on your head, the arrangement flips. Now the gas collects just below the entrance to your small intestine, while burping would result in a 'vomit burp' of liquid stomach contents. While you're unlikely to eat doing a handstand, meals taken semi-recumbent on the couch can shift your stomach's gas bubble, causing gas to pass preferentially into your small intestine rather than escaping as a burp.

Swallowed gases that make it to your small intestine have strayed beyond burp territory. The iron-clad sphincter between your stomach and small intestine will not permit backwards passage. The fate of these gases is perhaps surprising: they don't inflate you like a balloon or emerge later as a fart – they end up in your blood.

Gases are constantly moving in and out of your blood via a process called diffusion. Take oxygen, for example. It diffuses from inhaled air into your blood within your lungs, then diffuses out of your blood to fuel oxygen-hungry cells in your organs. Gases always diffuse from an area of higher concentration to an area of lower concentration. Gas diffusion happens in your guts too. Your intestinal walls are stuffed with blood vessels. The blood coursing through them absorbs nutrients from your food, but it also absorbs gases via diffusion. Swallowed air, just like inhaled air, contains 21 per cent oxygen. Swallowed oxygen will diffuse from your small intestines into your blood, just like inhaled oxygen diffuses into the blood flowing through your lungs. In a weird way, swallowing air offers an incredibly inefficient adjunct to blood oxygenation via breathing.

We haven't got very far trying to account for the 200 millilitres of gas that's always sitting in your gastrointestinal tract, since swallowed gas is mainly burped out and any gas that strays deeper into your guts ends up in your blood. A fraction of that 200 millilitres is hiding out as carbon dioxide in your small intestine. A fizz of CO_2 erupts like a bath bomb when your incoming acidic stomach contents are neutralised by those alkaline juices flowing from the sphincter of Oddi (bath bombs use citric acid rather than hydrochloric, but bicarbonate is the base in both reactions). Fat and protein digestion releases a few more carbon dioxide bubbles too. But none of this carbon dioxide makes it into your farts: it diffuses into your blood. If you're after gut gases, there's just one place you should look: your large intestine.

*

CT scanners use rotating X-ray machines to create cross-sectional images of your body. When a doctor looks at a CT scan of your abdomen, they can also see cross-sections of your liver and kidneys, but also cross-sections of the faeces sitting in your large intestine. Your doctor can also see your farts. They look like little black holes dotted around and mixed within your faeces. The odd thing is, *you* didn't make those farts. They're not even of mammalian origin. You can blame your flatulence on the bacteria living in your large intestine.

A one-gram fleck of faeces contains approximately 100 billion bacteria. One hundred *billion*. Half the dry weight of your stool is bacteria. The number of bacterial species in your large intestine runs into the thousands. These 'good' bacteria are handy critters to have around. They harmlessly take up real estate that disease-causing bacteria otherwise would. They also synthesise various vitamins including vitamin K (without which you couldn't form blood clots) and several B vitamins important for energy production and nerve function. In return for these favours, we allow the bacteria to live off the undigested food and fibre that make it to our large intestines.

If your small intestine fails to digest something you've eaten, the hungry mouths of your large intestine's bacterial zoo will ferment it into farts instead. Besides the embarrassment of flatulence, undigested food also causes diarrhoea by sucking water into your large intestine. Multiple upstream mishaps can result in undigested food hitting your large intestine. For example, fat digestion fails if your pancreas and gallbladder don't pitch in with their emulsifying, enzyme-rich liquids. Lactose, the sugar in milk, can go undigested if you lack lactase, the enzyme needed to break it down. If neither you nor your large intestinal bacteria completely digest something you've eaten, you'll see the remnants in the toilet bowl looking unsettlingly similar to how it appeared on your fork (vivid yellow corn kernels being the classic example).

Fibre is the catch-all term for the indigestible carbohydrates in plant foods like fruit, vegetables, seeds and grains. Herbivores can digest fibre, but the process is quite a palaver. Herbivores' intestines are at least 10 times their body length to provide enough gut transit time for nutrient extraction. Multiple stomachs and two rounds of digestion are often required. Ruminants – cud-chewing animals like cattle, sheep and deer – swallow their food, allow it to ferment in two of their four separate stomachs, then regurgitate the cud for a second chewing (hence why mentally brooding over a problem is called 'rumination', which comes from the Latin for 'chewing over again'). Even after chew number two, the grass remains too intact for ruminants' small intestines to extract its nutrients. Swallowed cud passes through a third and fourth stomach before finally it's ready for the small intestine (all 40 metres/130 feet of it, in cattle). While you're ruminating on that, consider the more practical approach taken by rabbits, who just eat their poo to allow a second round of fibre digestion.

Human guts can't physically digest fibre. Well, they can't anymore. Around 2.5 million years ago our hominin ancestors began eating calorie-packed meat. Maintaining the intestinal infrastructure to extract the scant calories from a mouthful of grass became a waste of energy. Evolution favoured shorter, more economical guts that let fibre pass straight through them, sparing their digestive efforts for more energy-dense meals, like the tenderloin of wild boar.

Although you can't digest fibre, the bacteria living in your large intestines can. The chemical reactions they use for digestion don't need oxygen: they extract energy from your digestive remnants via fermentation. Fermentation is a chemical reaction that produces gas. Bread rises thanks to carbon dioxide bubbles produced as yeast ferments the sugars in the dough. 'Holes' in Swiss cheese are trapped pockets of CO_2 released by *Proprionibacter shermani* bacteria as it ferments the lactic acid in milk (cheesemakers call the holes 'eyes'; if the fermentation process fails, the un-holey cheese is referred to as being 'blind'). Fermentation in your large intestine is responsible for those Swiss cheese 'holes' scattered through your faeces on that abdominal CT image: your farts.

Bacterial fermentation in your large intestine produces three main gases: hydrogen, carbon dioxide and methane. Despite its popular perception as 'the fart gas', only one in three people house methane-producing bacteria in their large intestines. Although nitrogen isn't produced by bacterial fermentation, it ends up in your large intestine because your blood dumps it there via diffusion. All up, hydrogen, carbon dioxide, nitrogen (and methane, for a third of the population) account for 99 per cent of your fart volume. The more fibre you eat, the more fermentation fodder you're providing the bacteria, and the more gas they'll make for you to release as farts.

Cast your mind back to that daily fart volume study. As well as measuring gas volumes, researchers performed gas composition analyses on the volunteers' emissions. As expected, farts collected during the beans-plus-whatever diet phase contained hydrogen, carbon dioxide and nitrogen (plus methane, in three of the ten volunteers). Farts on the fibre-free diet contained an unchanged volume of nitrogen, but only trace amounts of the other gases. Without fibre, the volunteers' large intestinal bacteria had nothing to ferment into hydrogen, carbon dioxide or methane. The only fart gas left was nitrogen, whose diffusion into the large intestine from the blood is unconnected to fibre intake. You'll recall that the fibre-free diet caused fart volume to reduce to just one-third: the missing two-thirds were those gases – hydrogen, CO_2 and sometimes methane – usually produced by bacterial fermentation.

So, we've accounted for 99 per cent of the gases in your farts, but it's the remaining one percent of gases that give your farts their most notable characteristic: foul smell.

A fart's stench, like the smell of bad breath, is predominantly due to sulfur-containing compounds like hydrogen sulfide. Other stinky gases include skatole (also found in low concentrations in jasmine and orange blossoms), short-chain fatty acids, ammonia and volatile amines. A fart's smell differs according to what you feed your large intestinal bacteria. Eat more high-sulfur foods like eggs, cheese and cabbage and your gut bacteria will produce more sulfur-containing gas. A quiche packed with vegetables is a bad dinner choice for campers sharing a two-person tent.

Two fart gases are flammable: hydrogen and methane. Since fire is captivating and farts are taboo, igniting farts is a timeless form of entertainment. The subject, usually intoxicated, will hold a lighter to their rear end and release some fermentation gases. The colour of the resultant jet of flame can tell you about the composition of the fart. Blue flames indicate the presence of methane: the subject belongs to the third of humans with methane-producing bacteria in their large intestine. Yellow or orange flames denote hydrogen ignition, the same reaction that caused the Hindenburg disaster (but in this case, with added smell). Oh, the humanity.

If you're ever reprimanded for a particularly offensive fart, your defence may be that *you* didn't produce it – the bacteria in your gut did.

SUMMARY: Burps represent the liberation of swallowed air from your stomach. Fibre fermentation by bacteria in your large intestine produces gas, which you release from your anus as farts.

AND ALSO …

Fatal farts

Diathermy is a surgical technique that uses an electric current to cut tissue or cauterise (burn closed) small blood vessels to stop bleeding. During colonoscopies, doctors use diathermy to remove polyps and take tissue samples. Colonic gas explosions have occurred when sparks from a diathermy device ignited fermentation gases. In 1979, a patient died when one such gas explosion burst open their large intestine:

> … there was an explosion which was audible in the endoscopy room, the patient jerked upwards off the endoscopy table, and the colonoscope was completely ejected … In spite of emergency surgery with transfusion of 45 units of blood, uncontrollable haemorrhage persisted from multiple bleeding points, and the patient died.[2]

The tragic case led to a change in colonoscopy procedures. The large intestine is now routinely inflated with a non-flammable gas (usually carbon dioxide or air) at the start of the colonoscopy. This inert gas dilutes the concentration of any flammable fermentation gases to below the levels required for ignition.

... and non-fatal farts

If you hold in a fart, it will just wait in your rectum until you're in the loo (or an empty elevator). Chronic fart repression can cause abdominal discomfort due to the trapped gas but doesn't pose any serious health risks. Roman emperor Claudius was not aware of this fact. According to Roman historian Suetonius, Claudius:

> ... considered passing an edict, by which he would give licence to farting at dinner, because he had heard of a man who had nearly killed himself by holding it in for shame.[3]

Permission to use the term 'anal cushions'

A trio of marshmallow-like skin pillows sits within your anal canal. When your anal sphincters squeeze, the pressure squashes the pillows together to prevent leakage. Your three anal cushions (yes, that's their anatomical name) are spongy due to their stuffing: juicy veins. If the anal cushions experience upstream pressure from chronic constipation or pregnancy, for example, they sag and droop from the anal canal. Enlarged anal cushions are called haemorrhoids. Due to their veiny contents, haemorrhoids bleed easily. The word haemorrhoids comes from the Greek *haima* (blood) and *rhoia* (flow). Other unwanted flowing fluids share that suffix include diarrhoea ('through flow'), steatorrhoea ('fat flow'; to describe the greasy stools of people with fat malabsorption), rhinorrhoea ('nose flow'; a runny nose) and menorrhoea ('moon flow'; bleeding during a period, 'moon' referring to their monthly frequency). Gonorrhoea literally means 'seed flow': the profusions of pus leaking from the penis were once thought to be semen ('seed' referring to the sperm within it). Gonorrhoea's nickname – 'the clap' – derives from the historical treatment of clapping one's hands along the penis to expel the pus. The preferred modern treatment is antibiotics.

And you thought *you* had trouble with gas

In 1886, American military surgeon Nicholas Senn pumped six litres (1.5 gallons) of gas up his rectum. He was attempting to demonstrate the safety of a technique he had invented to identify holes in the gastrointestinal tract caused by gunshot wounds. Senn often treated soldiers who had been shot in the abdomen. If the bullet had dodged their gastrointestinal tract, they didn't need urgent surgery. But it was a different story if faeces were leaking into the soldier's abdomen through a bullet hole in his intestines. Neither symptoms nor physical examination could determine if the bullet had pierced the soldier's guts. Senn's solution was simple: pump gas up the injured soldier's rectum and see if it hissed out from the abdominal wound. Senn began his experiments on dogs. The poor creatures were strapped to a table, anaesthetised, then shot in the abdomen with a 32-calibre revolver. Immediately after firing, hydrogen gas was pumped up their rectum. If the bullet had punctured the dog's gut, the gas would gush out the bullet wound. Senn would confirm that the gas was hydrogen by setting fire to it (he optimistically suggested that the flame would also sterilise the wound). If the bullet had missed the gut, the dog would just become very bloated from the rectally pumped gas. Senn's six-litre self-experimentation proved that humans, like dogs, could survive the gas inflation procedure even without a bullet wound to permit decompression. Senn explained how during his ordeal:

> ... colicky pains were experienced, which increased as insufflation advanced, and only ceased after all the gas had escaped, which was the case only after an hour and a half. When the intestines and the stomach had become fully distended the feeling of distention was distressing and was attended by a sensation of faintness which caused a profuse clammy perspiration. A great deal of the gas escaped by eructation [burping], which was followed by great relief.[4]

Senn's technique was used with some success but became obsolete when X-rays became widely available (battlefield X-rays were first used in 1897 during the Balkan War). A quick X-ray or two could instantly locate a bullet within an injured soldier – having punctured his gastrointestinal tract or otherwise – without requiring him to drop his pants.

ENDNOTES

1   Jeffries, S. Whip Hand. *The Guardian* (8 April 2006). https://www. theguardian.com/sport/2006/apr/08/horseracing.crimebooks
2   Bigard, M.A. et al. Fatal colonic explosion during colonoscopic polypectomy. *Gastroenterology*, 77 (6), 1307-10 (1979).
3   Suetonius, Divus Claudius 32.
4   Pilcher, J. E. Senn on the diagnosis of gastro-intestinal perforation by the rectal insufflation of hydrogen gas. *Annals of Surgery*, 8, 190–204 (1888).

URINARY UPSETS

To relieve yourself, pass water, spend a penny, have a piss, slash, tinkle, whizz, leak or number one. Call it what you will.

Urine was the first bodily fluid to be scientifically examined. This is perhaps to be expected: it's the most readily accessible liquid that your body produces. The technique of uroscopy – peering at a patient's pee for diagnostic purposes – is recorded in the clay tablets of Sumerian and Babylonian physicians from over 6000 years ago. For millennia (until about 300 years ago, in fact) uroscopy was a doctor's primary investigative tool. Urine was hailed as a divine fluid that offered a window into the inner workings of the body. Before stethoscopes, blood tests and CT scanners, physicians didn't have a lot of evidence on which to base their diagnoses. Examining the two litres (half a gallon) of fluid that flowed from their patient's body each day seemed like a logical way of deducing disorders upstream (as it were).

Around 400 BC, Hippocrates declared that: 'No other organ system or organ of the human body provides so much information by its excretion as does the urinary system.'[1] Urine, he believed, was a filtrate of the four humours: blood, black bile, yellow bile and phlegm (he was 25 per cent right: urine is a filtrate of blood). In his book *Aphorisms*, Hippocrates made diagnostic comments based on urine's colour ('when the urine is transparent and white, it is bad'), consistency and sediment ('thick urine' containing bran-like particles means that 'the bladder has scabies'), and odour ('a heavy smell' is suggestive of 'ulceration of the bladder').[2]

Hippocrates limited his deductions to problems with the kidneys and the bladder. But by the Middle Ages, physicians began making more ambitious inferences from the qualities of their patients' urine. Nearly every disease was reportedly associated with some specific change in the urine. Gilles de Corbeil, physician to the French royals around the start of the 13th century, included some of these diagnostic tips in *On Urines*, a 352-verse poem intended as a mnemonic for students of uroscopy:

- 'A large quantity of urine, darkened by black cloudiness ... and accompanied by poor hearing and insomnia, portends a flux of blood from the nose' (no, it doesn't; see *Nosebleeds*, page 100).
- Urine that is 'livid near the surface' may suggest 'an ailment of the womb', 'a defect of the lungs', 'pain in the joints' or 'falling sickness' (your guess is as good as mine).
- 'Dancing' or 'overmuch coitus' may result in urine that is 'wine coloured' or 'blue-black'.
- 'Thin urine, white in colour' is indicative of at least a dozen complaints including epilepsy, dropsy, intoxication, dizziness, 'chill of liver' and death (in my experience, absence of a pulse is a more reliable indicator of death than any changes in urine). If the patient is old, however, the interpretation differed: 'it is a sign of debility or childishness'.[3]

By the 14th century, the practice of uroscopy had become as convoluted as de Corbeil's poetry. Urine samples had to be examined in a specially designed glass flask called a matula. Matulas were shaped like bladders in the belief that diagnostic accuracy was enhanced by allowing the urine sample to conform to a familiar-shaped vessel. Every respectable physician owned a matula, which he would pensively hold up to the light to scrutinise his patient's liquid offerings. Matulas were a badge of honour, a symbol of the profession much like a stethoscope or white coat is today. Early matulas were divided into four sections: urine in the uppermost section corresponded to diseases of the head, then sequentially the chest, abdomen and bladder. Before long matulas were manufactured with 11 sections to cover more of the organs in each body cavity. Matula madness climaxed in the 15th century when a human body-shaped matula, divided into 24 sections, hit the market.

As faith in uroscopy grew, some doctors viewed meeting their patients as optional. Instead, they would prognosticate based solely on urine samples sent to them by their patients. This was a mutually agreeable arrangement. Physicians could churn through (and charge for) far more 'urine-only consults' than in-person house calls per day. Patients preferred uroscopy too: offering their urine up for examination was far more discreet than stripping nude and lying on a table, a matter particularly important to women.

By the 16th century, belief in urine's portentous power had spiralled out of control. Translations of medical manuscripts, previously only available in Latin, made uroscopy accessible to the masses. Untrained quacks claimed to be able to 'read' a person's urine to predict their future, a practice known as uromancy. Respectable physicians sought to distance themselves from these 'piss prophets' as they became known. Thomas Linacre, who founded the Royal College of Physicians in London in 1518, ridiculed doctors who were 'too ready to carry about the patient's urine, expecting they would be told all things from the mere speculation of it' and sarcastically suggested that a patient's urine was about as useful a diagnostic tool as their shoe.[4]

The final nail in the coffin came in 1637, when physician Thomas Brian published *The Pisse Prophet*, a scathing take-down of the increasingly unscientific approach to uroscopy. Brian mocked 'the pisse-pot science, used by all those (whether quacks and empiricks, or other methodical physicians) who pretend knowledge of diseases, by the urine, in giving judgement of the same.'[5] He expressed dismay at the way some doctors were avoiding interacting with patients, substituting uromancy for taking a patient's history and physically examining them: '... it were fare better for the physician to see his patient once than to view his urine twenty times.' As Europe entered the Age of Enlightenment, uroscopy fell out of vogue, dismissed as voodoo pseudoscience. The golden age of urine was over.

*

To be fair, the piss prophets did get some things right. Under very specific circumstances, urine can be used to predict your future (like if you're going to have a baby) and reveal truths about your past (such as if you ate beetroot on a poppy seed bagel for breakfast). Urine is certainly not a 'divine fluid', but it is quite a handy diagnostic tool, as we will soon discover. But first we must meet the urine makers: the kidneys.

Kidneys resemble kidney beans in colour and shape. Each kidney is about the size of your fist. Statistically speaking, you've probably got two kidneys: one on either side of your spine tucked neatly behind your lower ribs. But of all the organs, kidneys show the most variability in number and location. For example, some people have both kidneys on one side of their body. Others have one kidney in the usual spot, plus one adventurous ectopic kidney down in their pelvis, or even nestled against a lung in their chest. One in 500 people have a single 'horseshoe kidney', where both organs are fused at the base into a U-shaped lump. Some people have one kidney on one side, and two on the other (bringing their tally to three), or even a pair of kidneys on both sides (four kidneys in total). Usually these anatomical quirks cause no problems and are identified incidentally upon having a CT scan of your abdomen for some other reason. While it's nice to have a spare (or several spares), you only really need one kidney to survive, which is why you can donate a kidney to a relative in need and continue your life unscathed (the same cannot be said of heart donors).

Whatever number of kidneys you have, each kidney does the same thing: it filters your blood. Your kidneys remove excess water, waste products and unwanted chemicals from the blood that's constantly flowing through them. The percolated product – urine – persistently drips out of each kidney down a pair of 30-centimetre-long (12-inch-long) tubes called ureters into your bladder. At a convenient moment you eject this fluid via a single tube called the urethra. A woman's urethra is about four centimetres (1.5 inches) long. Men, whose urethra needs to traverse the length of their penis, have urethras that are about 20 centimetres (eight inches) long. This length discrepancy is the main reason why women get so many more bladder infections than men: it's much easier for disease-causing bacteria in your environment to shimmy up a short tube than a long one.

You'll feel a mild urge to wee when there's about 150 millilitres (5 fl oz) of urine in your bladder. Discomfort sets in at 400 millilitres (13.5 fl oz). Bladder rupture from 'holding on' is exceedingly rare: you'll just wet your pants at a bladder volume of around 600 millilitres (20 fl oz). Legend has it that Danish astronomer Tycho Brahe (1546–1601) died after his bladder burst during a banquet. Apparently, he was too polite to excuse himself to urinate. It's more likely that he died from kidney failure, or perhaps mercury poisoning at the hand of his assistant Johannes Kepler. Car accidents, rather than pathologically good table manners, account for most cases of burst bladders. The seat belt strap exerts hefty compressive forces on the lower abdomen, just over the bladder, as the car slams to a halt.

Immediately after leaving the bladder, a man's urethra traverses his walnut-sized prostate gland. Well, at least it was walnut-sized in his 20s. Prostates predictably plump up with age. After his

50th birthday, a man's chance of having an enlarged prostate is roughly equal to his age: 60 per cent of 60-year-olds have enlarged prostates; make it to 90 and there's a 90 per cent of having an enlarged prostate. As the prostate grows it gradually compresses the urethra running through it. The urine stream might dwindle to a weak dribble. Initiating urination can require straining akin to passing a bowel movement. Incomplete bladder emptying can cause maddening repeated toilet trips, particularly overnight.

Surgery to core out the prostate can be life-changing for a man with an enlarged, urethra-strangling prostate. Particularly pudgy prostates can completely choke the urethra. Excruciating pain soon sets in as the bladder balloons with trapped urine. Poking a catheter up the urethra – carefully threading it along the penis, through the prostate's iron grip and into the bladder – can drain the accumulated urine and provide instant relief. I once performed this procedure on a nonagenarian who was so grateful that he cried and attempted to award me the Victoria Cross (he thought it was 1945: the pain had rendered him profoundly delirious).

*

A staggering volume of blood flows through your kidneys each day. Every time your heart beats, one quarter of the blood it pumps out heads straight to your kidneys for scrubbing. Healthy kidneys can filter 120 millilitres (4 fl oz) of blood per minute, which equates to about 170 litres (45 gallons) per day. That's correct: every 24 hours your two little kidneys filter a bathtub's worth of blood. How much waste fluid – urine – does that generate? The metric system makes this calculation easy. Take your weight in kilograms, change the units to millilitres, and that's about the volume of urine your kidneys make per hour. So, an 80-kilogram (176 pound) person makes about 80 millilitres (3 fl oz) of urine an hour, or about 1.9 litres (half a gallon) per day.

Urine – like cucumbers, jellyfish and cheap perfume – is mainly water: 95 per cent water in fact. The remaining five per cent comprises dissolved debris from your blood. Excess sodium, chloride, calcium and potassium ions are removed from your body via your urine. Metabolic waste products end up in your urine too; the junk by-products generated by your body's constant chemical reactions. Flexing your arm, for example, requires muscle cells in your biceps to perform energy-producing reactions. Creatinine, a waste product of those reactions, seeps into your bloodstream for your kidneys to filter out into your urine. Your body's cells are constantly dying and being replaced. Dead cells are broken down and scavenged for parts which can be recycled. Many of the remaining waste products end up flushed down the toilet. A red blood cell, for example, will do laps of your body for 120 days before it dies. The valuable iron will be extracted from the cell's corpse for reuse. Urobilin, a chemical produced as the red blood cell's haemoglobin is broken down, gives urine its yellow hue (see *Bruising*, page 246).

If there's not enough water in your urine to keep the filtered waste dissolved, the waste products will crystalise into hard lumps: kidney stones. Sometimes the crystallisation results in an enormous antler-like structure within the kidney, known as a staghorn calculus. Kidney stones are common: 19 percent of men and nine per cent of women will be diagnosed with one by the age of 70. About 80 to 90 per cent of kidney stones contain calcium. People who consume high-purine foods and beverages (like liver, sardines, and beer) are prone to developing stones made from uric acid, a by-product of purine breakdown. Struvite stones, which contain magnesium, ammonia and phosphate, can form after bladder infections.

Once a kidney stone forms there's only one way out: down the ureter, into the bladder and out the urethra. The excruciating pain as the jagged rock slowly scrapes down the 30-centimetre-long (12 inches long) ureter is considered one of the most severe pains a human can experience, on par with cluster headaches (see *Headache*, page 16). I once treated a patient who had experienced both the ejection of a kidney stone and a set of twins from her body. She didn't pause when I asked her which was more painful: 'The stone!' Most stones under four millimetres (0.16 inches) will eventually pass spontaneously but can take up to a month to scrape their way out. Larger stones may need to be fished out surgically or shattered into gravel using high-energy ultrasound shock waves fired at your flanks.

You can hasten the passage of a kidney stone by keeping hydrated, or by riding on a roller coaster, as a 2016 study showed.[6] Urologist Professor David Wartinger was inspired to test the roller coaster technique after a patient alleged that a stone had popped out after a ride on the Big Thunder Mountain Railroad at Florida's Walt Disney World. A true scientist, Wartinger flew to Florida with a pocketful of fake kidney stones and a plastic model of a kidney and ureter. Twenty times, Wartinger loaded the kidney with stones and accompanied it, safely tucked in a backpack, on the coaster. He reported: 'The model was subjected to sharp turns and quick drops during the ride, which lasted 2 minutes and 30 seconds.' He discovered that the teeth-rattling vibrations induced in a rear seat position were most effective at hurrying the stone along the ureter: 63.89 per cent of stones jiggled free when the model was placed in the back carriage compared to just 16.67 per cent in a smoother front carriage position. For patients with kidney stones that just won't budge, Disney World really is 'Where dreams come true'.

*

What you eat influences your urine's composition. Digesting the protein in a chicken breast, for example, releases the waste chemical urea into your blood. The more protein you eat, the more urea your kidneys will have to scrub from your blood. Tofu, eggs, and cottage cheese are popular high-protein foods that will cause a blood urea spike for your kidneys to clean up. Blood itself, however, is a less popular protein-rich food. While you're unlikely to voluntarily eat blood (unless you're a black pudding fan), you may unwittingly end up with blood in your stomach if you've got a bleeding stomach ulcer, for example. As the haemorrhaged blood passes through your digestive tract, your intestines will digest the protein in it just like any other high-protein meal. The resulting surge in blood urea levels, which can be measured with a blood test, provides doctors with a very useful clue that there's internal bleeding going on. Any patient clutching their stomach in pain with a sky-high blood urea level is presumed to be bleeding into their gastrointestinal tract until proven otherwise. (An alternative explanation is that the stomach ache and high blood urea are due to a recent overindulgence at a steakhouse – hopefully this differential is excluded based on the patient's history.)

Various things you can snort, smoke or inject into your veins can end up in your urine. Urine drug tests for athletes are based on the fact that your kidneys will percolate breakdown products of anabolic steroids into your urine. Metabolites of cocaine, cannabis, benzodiazepines, and opiates like heroin, morphine and codeine all end up in your urine too. Eating poppy seeds will give you a positive urine drug test for opioids for the next 24 hours. American prisons don't serve any foods containing poppy seeds in order to avoid confusion over false positive urine screens for opioids. Prisoners granted day leave must sign a form agreeing to eschew poppy seeds during their outing, preventing them from pleading 'I just ate a bagel, sir' as an excuse for failing the mandatory urine drug test upon their return.

Under the right circumstances, urine can come in any colour of the rainbow. Beeturia describes the alarming red-tinged urine experienced by about 10 per cent of the population after eating beetroot. Rifampicin, a drug used to treat tuberculosis, colours bodily fluids including tears, sweat and urine a vibrant orange. Patients prescribed rifampicin are warned not to wear white

T-shirts (to avoid orange sweat stains) or use contact lenses (their tears will dye the lenses orange). High-dose vitamin B supplements will turn your urine the colour of a modern tennis ball (before 1972 tennis balls were white; the shift to 'optic yellow' occurred because the fluorescent ball showed up better on colour TV). The bacterium *Pseudomonas aeruginosa* is an attractive shade of jade and will colour infected urine similarly. Michael Jackson died from an overdose of the anaesthetic propofol, a drug which can turn urine white, pink or green.

Methylene blue is a harmless dye used to label tissues during surgery. If ingested, it will be excreted in your urine. I once worked with a venerable surgeon who reminisced about a methylene blue-based prank he used to play on medical students. He'd carefully inject praline chocolates with the dye, then leave the chocolates prominently positioned in the surgical wing's common room. Ravenous cash-strapped medical students would devour the spiked chocolates for breakfast. Come lunchtime, the surgeon and his chums would loiter around the urinals to watch the students panic upon passing bright blue urine.

Some people are born with genetic defects that mean they can't break down certain amino acids (the building blocks of proteins) in the food they eat. The partially metabolised waste products accumulate in their blood and are filtered into their urine, often giving it a characteristic colour or smell. There are hundreds of these so-called 'inherited disorders of metabolism'. Some of them have self-explanatory names like 'maple syrup urine disease' (referring to the urine's sweet odour) or 'blue-diaper syndrome'. Others have less catchy names but highly memorable urine smells such as swimming pool-like (seen in the disorder called hawkinsinuria), cabbage-like (typical of tyrosinemia), fishy (trimethylaminuria), mousy (phenylketonuria) or reminiscent of sweaty feet (isovaleric acidemia).

Peering at your urine like a medieval uroscopist can sometimes identify kidney diseases. Your kidneys are very selective in what they filter out of your blood. Healthy kidneys would never remove precious red blood cells, protein, components of your immune system (like white blood cells) or glucose from your blood. If any of these substances do end up in your urine, it's a sign that your kidneys aren't working properly. Here's what to look out for. Red blood cells will make your urine look red; protein-filled urine will froth furiously and form a head on the toilet bowl water to rival a well-tapped glass of Guinness. White blood cells make urine look like cloudy apple juice. Urine with glucose in it, seen in people with uncontrolled diabetes, looks normal, but tastes sickly sweet (not that I'd recommend taking a sip). This is because when blood glucose levels get very high, the excess glucose overwhelms the kidneys' filtration system and ends up in the urine. The proper medical name for diabetes is *diabetes mellitus*, meaning 'go through sweet'. Physician Thomas Willis coined the term in 1674 after bravely drinking a diabetic's urine and describing it as 'wonderfully sweet as if it were imbued with honey or sugar'.[7] Willis wasn't the first to make this observation: ancient Hindu physicians around 6 BC were aware that some people (diabetics, in retrospect) had sweet urine which attracted black ants.

*

To avoid death, your blood's acidity and its concentrations of dissolved ions must be strictly controlled. Minor deviations in blood chemistry can be lethal because your body's cells only work within a very narrow chemical window. For example, your blood's pH must remain between 7.35 and 7.45 to avoid stupor, seizures, and death. Your kidneys are responsible for keeping your blood chemistry on an even keel by carefully juggling what they remove from your blood. What you eat has essentially zero impact on the composition of your blood. You can snack on a sack of salt, down a bottle of vinegar or eat spoonfuls of baking soda and your kidneys will perform the required extractions to keep your blood's composition stable. The notion of eating foods to 'make your body more alkaline', for example, is as unscientific as uromancy.

While on urine-based myths, let me bust the big one: you don't need to drink eight glasses of water a day, you only need to drink when you feel thirsty. Needing to make such a bleedingly obvious statement is testament to the marketing prowess of bottled water companies. An early appearance of the 'eight glasses' myth features in a 1974 book *Nutrition for Good Health*, co-authored by American nutritionists Frederick Stare and Margaret McWilliams.[8] The duo recommended a water intake of 'somewhere around 6 to 8 glasses per 24 hours' with two disclaimers: water intake is 'usually well regulated' by your sense of thirst, and a reminder that the foods you eat contribute significantly to your daily fluid quota. For instance, a 100-gram (3.5 ounces) dollop of yoghurt or mashed potato holds 80 millilitres (2.7 fl oz) of water. Eat a 250-gram (8.8 grams) punnet of strawberries and you've just 'drunk' 225 millilitres (7.6 fl oz) of water. Even seemingly bone-dry foods contain water, like corn flakes (four per cent water) and potato chips (two percent water). Alas, the nutritionists' disclaimers dropped off the radar and the 'eight glasses' advice became fact, incorporated into national health guidelines and religiously obeyed by water bottle-toting gym junkies to this day. It's a myth. Delete the 'hydration app' from your smartphone and just drink when you're thirsty like every other animal on Earth does.

Gulping down extra water when you're not thirsty will not 'help' your kidneys any more than beating your chest like Tarzan will 'help' your heart pump. Swallowed water is absorbed through the lining of your intestines into your bloodstream. If you drink more water than your body requires, your kidneys will just extract the extra water from your blood (i.e. make more urine) to keep your blood chemistry stable – to a point.

Rapidly gulping gallons of fluid will quickly dilute the salts in your blood. Even working at maximal capacity, your kidneys will take a while to remove the excess water to return your blood's salt concentrations to normal. In the meantime, your brain can bloat with fluid. When your increasingly swollen brain becomes too big to fit inside your skull, it will squeeze through the hole at the base of your cranium – resulting in instant death (see *Headache*, page 10).

Deaths from accidently drinking too much – water intoxication – have been reported among people zealously rehydrating after a bout of gastroenteritis, marathon runners incessantly sipping during a race, people participating in water-drinking competitions run by radio stations, and those with psychogenic polydipsia, a psychiatric condition where the patient experiences strong urges to drink:

> On the evening before her death, she began compulsively drinking water in vast quantities, estimated at between 30 and 40 glasses, and this was interspersed with episodes of vomiting. She became hysterical and also distressed, shouting that she had not drunk enough water. She declined medical attention but continued to drink water after she had gone to bed. She later fell asleep and died some time later.[9]

*

The only thing you should do with your urine is flush it down the toilet. Don't bathe in it, use it as a throat gargle, or pour it on battle wounds or sliced-off noses. This advice is not offered without reason: eminent figures throughout history have promoted all of those activities as treatments for an array of maladies. Pliny the Elder (23–79 AD) endorsed the application of fresh urine as a cure for 'sores, burns, affections of the anus, chaps and scorpion stings'.[10] English physician and cleric William Bullein (1515–1576) swore by a skin-clearing face wash of 'strong vinegar, milk and the urine of a boy'.[11] French surgeon Ambroise Paré (1510–1590) suggested that itching eyelids could be alleviated by dousing them with the patient's urine after it had been 'kept all night in a barber's basin'.[12] Thomas Willis (1621–1675), of diabetes mellitus coining fame, advised a young woman to drink her own urine to counter the 'extreme sourness' in her throat.[11]

Frank Zappa's 1974 hit song 'Don't Eat the Yellow Snow' offers practical medical advice in its chorus, in which Zappa chants the song's title. Indeed, there are no benefits to eating frozen urine or drinking it fresh 'whil'st 'tis yet warm' as Robert Boyle, known as the father of chemistry, advocated.[13] You're just insulting your kidneys by forcing them to refilter the waste products they'd already diligently extracted from your blood. Nevertheless, urinobibes (people who drink their own urine) claim that the practice promotes good health.

American author J. D. Salinger, best known for his 1951 classic *The Catcher in the Rye*, was a urinobibe. So was Morarji Desai, the fourth Prime Minister of India, who lived to be 99 (in spite of, not because of, the urine drinking). And you were a urinobibe too, when you were in your mother's womb. Look at an ultrasound of a foetus and you'll see it swimming in amniotic fluid. Initially that liquid comes from the mother's body. But when the foetus's kidneys start working at about 11 weeks of gestation, its urine begins contributing to that fluid. By 20 weeks, the amniotic fluid is mostly foetal urine. As well as providing a buffer from maternal belly bumps and knocks, the foetus inhales and drinks its urine to help its lungs and gastrointestinal tract to develop. A woman's 'waters breaking' denotes the rupture of this urine bag, heralding the imminent birth of the baby. This is perhaps the only time when being doused in urine may be a cause for excitement, unless you're a urolagniac: a person who finds sexual gratification in being urinated on.

SUMMARY: Your kidneys filter your blood to remove excess water and waste chemicals to form a liquid called urine. Don't drink it. Drink water instead, but only if you're thirsty.

AND ALSO ...

Astronomical embarrassment

Wetting oneself is undignified at the best of times, let alone when you're wearing a space suit while strapped inside a rocket. Launch delays on 5 May 1961 meant that astronaut Alan Shepard spent eight long bladder-stretching hours on the launchpad. He no doubt regretted his liquid breakfast of orange juice and coffee. Shepard finally radioed: 'Man, I gotta pee'.[14] Mission control had no choice but to advise him to wet himself. They kindly cut off his electrical biosensors to prevent urine-electrocution. As the pee pooled in his lower back, a relieved Shepard joked: 'I'm a wetback now'. Suffice it to say that all future missions incorporated a urine bag and drainage system into the space suit.

We all wee for 21 seconds

In 2013, researchers armed with high-speed video cameras visited Zoo Atlanta to film various mammals urinating, seeking to identify the relationship between an animal's size and how long it took to empty its bladder.[15] Their results were succinctly summarised by the title of their paper: 'Law of Urination: all mammals empty their bladders over the same duration'. Despite larger mammals having bigger bladders with more urine to release than smaller mammals, bladder emptying took 21 seconds, on average, across all the mammals filmed. The explanation comes down to urethral anatomy. Larger mammals have longer urethras, allowing them to achieve stronger urine jets due to higher gravitational forces and flow speeds. Smaller mammals have far less urine to release, but the high surface tension in their piddly urethras limits their urine release to slow, single drops.

Urine for a baby in about nine months

Urine was central to the first documented pregnancy test, recorded in an ancient Egyptian medical papyrus written around 1350 BC. Rather than wee on a stick and wait for lines to appear, the woman would 'water' barley and wheat seeds every day with her urine until one seed germinated. 'If the barley grows [first], it means a male child. If the wheat grows [first], it means a female child. If both do not grow, she will not bear at all.'[16] The gender logic is inexplicable, but the test had a 50 per cent hit rate just by chance. Modern pregnancy tests work by detecting a hormone called human chorionic gonadotropin (hCG) in a woman's urine. When a fertilised egg implants in a woman's uterus, it starts pumping out hCG. This hCG enters the woman's bloodstream and is filtered by the kidneys into her urine, ready to be detected by a pregnancy test. In 2018, IKEA produced magazine advertisements for a crib with the caption: 'peeing on this ad may change your life'. The page doubled as a pregnancy test. If a woman had hCG in her urine, weeing on the marked area would reveal a message telling her she was pregnant, accompanied by a 50 per cent discount coupon for the featured crib.

ENDNOTES

1   Kouba, E. et al. Uroscopy by Hippocrates and Theophilus: Prognosis Versus Diagnosis. *The Journal of Urology*, 177 (1), 50-52 (2007).

2   Hippocrates. *Aphorisms*. Translated by Adams, F. (1849). http://classics.mit.edu/Hippocrates/aphorisms.html.

3   Wallis, F. *Medieval Medicine: A Reader*. University of Toronto Press (2010).

4   Connor, H. Medieval Uroscopy and Its Representation on Misericords – Part 1: Uroscopy. *Clinical Medicine*, 1 (6), 507–509 (2001).

5   Brian, T. *The Pisse-prophet, Or, Certaine Pisse-pot Lectures: Wherein Are Newly Discovered the Old Fallacies, Deceit, and Jugling of the Pissepot Science, Used By All Those (whether Quacks and Empiricks, or Other Methodicall Physicians) Who Pretend Knowledge of Diseases, By the Urine, in Giving Judgement of the Same*. London, Thrale (1637).

6   Mitchell, M. A. & Wartinger, D. D. Validation of a Functional Pyelocalyceal Renal Model for the Evaluation of Renal Calculi Passage While Riding a Roller Coaster. *The Journal of the American Osteopathic Association*, 116, 647-652 (2016).

7   Feudtner, C. *Bittersweet: Diabetes, Insulin, and the Transformation of Illness*. University of North Carolina Press (2004).

8   Stare, F. & McWilliams, M. *Nutrition for Good Health*. Plycon Press (1974).

9   Farrell D. J. & Bower, L. Fatal water intoxication. *Journal of Clinical Pathology*, 56 (10), 803-804 (2003),

10 Pliny the Elder. *Natural History*. Translated by Rackham, H. Harvard University Press (1949).

11 Sugg, R. *Mummies, Cannibals and Vampires: the History of Corpse Medicine from the Renaissance to the Victorians*. Taylor & Francis (2012).

12 Johnson, T. & Paré, A. *The Works of that Famous Chirurgion Ambrose Parey: Translated Out of Latine and Compared with the French*. United Kingdom, Th. Cotes and R. Young (1634).

13 Boyle, R. *Medicinal experiments or A collection of choice remedies for the most part simple, and easily prepared*. London, Smith (1692).

14 Pappas, C. *One Giant Leap: Iconic and Inspiring Space Race Inventions that Shaped History*. Lyons Press (2019).

15 Yang, P. J. et al. Law of Urination: all mammals empty their bladders over the same duration. *Fluid Dynamics,* arXiv: 1310.3737 (2013).

16 Burstein, J. & Braunstein G. D. Urine pregnancy tests from antiquity to the present. *Early Pregnancy,* 1, 288–96 (1995).

SKIN

BRUISING

Gaudy and long-lasting, bruises are the musical theatre of the skin.

I once assisted in an operation on an elderly woman who had fallen over Monty, her Maltese Shih Tzu. From hip to knee, the outside of her right thigh was black with bruising. There was no way that the bruise would be resolved without surgery. The surgical technique in this situation is to slice open the skin covering the bruise and scrape out the clotted blood. The lead surgeon was a man with hands the size of hubcaps: the incision would have had to be enormous to accommodate them. As this dawned on him, I grinned and waggled my hands to demonstrate my scrawny wrists. Over the next half hour, I proceeded to evacuate several jars' worth of bloody, jam-like material. Her wound healed magnificently, and she was back with Monty within the week.

Bruises are puddles of blood released from crushed blood vessels, trapped under the skin. You've probably never given much thought to your blood vessels. Consider that your body is plumbed with sufficient vasculature to wrap around the circumference of the Earth. Twice! And another half again! Frankly, this seems excessive. But when you consider that each of your 37 trillion or so cells needs a tiny river of blood nearby, your internal plumbing seems more reasonable. The blood giveth, and the blood taketh away. Cells suck up oxygen and nutrients from blood flowing in nearby vessels. Cells also dump their waste into the blood for disposal, such as carbon dioxide (which you exhale when the blood flows through your lungs) and other metabolic waste chemicals (which your liver breaks down, or your kidneys percolate into urine).

The room air you inhale is 21 per cent oxygen but your exhaled breath still contains a whopping 16 per cent oxygen. Yep, most of the oxygen you inhale is simply exhaled again. Your blood is so efficient at sucking oxygen out of the air that it becomes completely saturated with plenty of oxygen to spare. The unused oxygen in what you breathe out is why mouth-to-mouth resuscitation works: there's still enough oxygen in your breath to be helpful to a person who can't breathe for themselves. Conversely, blowing tobacco smoke up a dying patient's rectum is *not* an effective resuscitation technique. Physicians in the 18th century believed that rectally delivered smoke would 'warm the patient and stimulate the heart'. They were mistaken. In reality, the smoke would have just infused the stool that was sitting in the patient's rectum. Without chest compressions, the patient's heart would remain unstimulated and they would likely die, only to unceremoniously expel that smoky stool on the autopsy table. Indeed, cadavers often have a final bowel action as their anal sphincters relax after death. The sound of flatulence is commonplace in the mortuary as gases escape the corpses' bowels. A pale-faced nurse once claimed that a patient I had recently pronounced dead had 'come back to life' after she heard him emit a massive fart. I reassured her that flatulence was not a sign of life and that he was still definitely dead.

Your blood vessels form a closed circuit in your body. The blood leaving your heart is the same as the blood returning to it – it's just nutritionally deplete and carrying junk, like tourists returning from a cheap cruise holiday. This 'closed circuit' notion is the sort of thing that is obvious when you think about it but is easy to overlook unless directly considered (like the fact that 'Baa Baa Black Sheep', 'Twinkle Twinkle Little Star' and 'The Alphabet Song' are all the same tune with different lyrics). To form a single loop, all outgoing vessels – arbitrarily called arteries – must eventually turn back towards the heart. The incoming vessels are called veins. The critical vessels at the U-turn point (capillaries) are where bruises usually occur.

Let's take a quick trip around the circuit. Your heart ejects high-pressure oxygenated blood via the aorta, an artery the width of your thumb. It's shaped like a walking stick. It shoots up a few centimetres (about an inch), peaks at the level where your collarbones meet, plunges down to supply your guts then divides in two (one artery for each leg). Your aorta runs just in front of your spinal column, literally touching the vertebrae as it traverses your torso. In this position it's tucked safely away from most pointy weapons (unless you get stabbed in the back or shatter your spine and a sharp bone fragment pierces your aorta from behind).

Along its length your aorta gives off many branches. Each branch branches, then each of those branches also branches and eventually these successive divisions give rise to tributaries with walls just one cell wide: thin enough for oxygen and nutrients in your blood to move across that wall into neighbouring cells. These vessels are your capillaries. All of your organs – your skin, brain, liver, even the surfaces of your eyeballs (take a look in a mirror) – are laced with dense capillary networks.

Having offloaded oxygen and nutrients and become filled with waste, blood must return to the lungs to refresh. Capillaries merge to form veins, which in turn merge until one thick pipe delivers blood back into your heart. As opposed to your heart's single outflow tract (the aorta), you've got one inflow tract entering your heart from the north and another from the south (the superior and inferior *vena cava*, respectively). Pump! The blood does a lap around the lungs, swapping its carbon dioxide (as you exhale) for oxygen (as you inhale). Pump! Ahoy, back out to the body! An elegant, infinite cycle. Or, less romantically, a very finite cycle lasting 72.6 years for the average earthling born in 2019, according to the United Nation's latest statistics.[1]

If your heart stops, it's helpful to get someone to press firmly on your chest to force blood through the circuit. Chest compressions are a key part of cardiopulmonary resuscitation (CPR). You've got to press hard enough on the breastbone to squeeze the blood out of the heart lying just beneath it. When you release, blood naturally fills the heart's empty chambers, ready for you to squeeze it out again with the next compression. Junior doctors practise pumping the chests of rib-less mannequins with deceptively pliable rubber torsos. In real life, chests are stiff, and CPR is exhausting. You're probably not doing effective CPR unless you hear the patient's ribs cracking. If you happen to have direct access to the dying person's heart you can perform cardiac massage: frantically squeezing the heart like a stress ball to keep the flow going. The need for cardiac massage can arise if a patient's heart arrests during open heart surgery (as in the case of Princess Diana).

Most of your widest blood vessels are buried deep inside your body, reducing the risk of a paper cut leading to lethal haemorrhage. But there are a few anatomical sites where big vessels lie perilously close to your body's surface. Press your fingers to one side of your neck: that throbbing is your carotid artery, one of a pair of arteries running on either side of your neck that supply blood to your brain. 'Carotid' comes from the Greek *karotis* meaning 'to stupefy', since compressing these arteries can cause unconsciousness by temporarily depriving your brain of blood (take your fingers off now, please). Capitalising on this fact, police have historically used a technique called 'carotid restraint' to incapacitate people. From behind, the officer grabs the person in a headlock, holding their arm tightly bent around the suspect's neck to exert pressure over both carotids. Ideally the person is swiftly stupefied and stops resisting as they crumple to the ground. But held too long, 'carotid sleeper holds' can cause brain death, trigger fatal heart rhythms or simply strangle the person if their trachea is accidentally squashed rather than just the carotids.

For this reason, most authorities worldwide have banned 'lateral vascular neck restraint', as it is also euphemistically dubbed, as a detainment method.

If your carotid artery is accidentally sliced by a wayward sharp object, the first aid treatment is compression to stop the blood squirting out. This advice holds for all injuries involving bleeding. In 1989 ice hockey goalie Clint Malarchuk took a skate blade to the neck when an opponent, Steve Tuttle, slammed into his goal area. Malarchuk's right carotid artery was slashed open. Malarchuk later recounted in his autobiography:

> A stream gushed out with every beat of my heart ... I
> grabbed my neck, trying to keep the blood in, but it rushed
> between my fingers. It just kept coming. I slumped forward
> and it glugged out like a water fountain.[2]

Footage shows blood gushing from the 15 centimetre (6 inch) wound and pooling on the ice with shocking speed. The clearly disturbed commentator pleads: 'Oh, god! Oh, please take the camera off, don't even bring it over there, please!' Luckily, Jim Pizzutelli, a former US Army combat medic and athletic trainer for Malarchuk's team, was sitting ringside. Pizzutelli had the presence of mind to dash onto the rink and pinch Malarchuk's severed carotid to prevent him exsanguinating. It's said that 11 fans fainted, two suffered heart attacks and a trio of players vomited on the rink. Three hundred sutures and 1.5 litres (three pints) of transfused blood later, Malarchuk was still alive. Remarkably, he was playing again in just ten days.

Injuries in which the skin is sliced open allow blood to drip out of your body (or torrentially pour out, in Malarchuk's case). But whacking, crushing or twisting injuries don't necessarily break the skin. Blood still leaks from damaged blood vessels but is trapped under your skin. This entombed blood, as seen through the skin, is a bruise.

When patients present to the emergency department having collided with something, doctors refer to the situation as 'patient versus X'. For instance: 'pedestrian versus car' or 'squash ball versus eye' (squash balls and human eyes share almost the same dimensions. A well-aimed squash ball can rupture your eyeball and take its place in the newly vacated eye socket). A bruise from a low-impact injury (like shin versus coffee table) will show up within a few hours since the crushed capillaries are close to the surface. Injuries involving deeper structures (like ankle versus pothole) damage deeper, more voluminous veins. It takes a while for the leaked blood to track up to the skin's surface, so if you're looking for sympathy, wait until 24 hours post-injury to take any selfies.

Heat, pain, redness and swelling: these are the four features of inflammation. Roman scholar Celsus documented these signs about 2000 years ago in a catchy Latin rhyme: *calor, dolor, rubor, tumor.* The physician Galen added 'loss of function' – *functio laesa* – to the list a century afterwards. I suspect Celsus knew this was part of the inflammatory response, but just omitted it because it messed up the rhyme. Tissue damage from any cause – bruise, burn, boil, bee sting – releases an eye-wateringly complex cascade of inflammatory chemicals to achieve tissue repair. The chemicals increase blood flow to the injured area, accounting for your freshly sprained ankle being hot and red. The surge of blood brings a wave of reparative cells which leak into the injured tissue, causing your ankle to swell. Other inflammatory chemicals activate local nerve endings to cause pain which renders your ankle impossible to walk on. This loss of function forces you to keep still, allowing time for uninterrupted healing.

Although your ego may be irreparably bruised after a public faceplant, there are a few steps you can take to minimise the size of your impending ankle bruise. Blood, like maple syrup, flows slower when it's colder. Applying ice to a bruised area slows the rate that blood leaks from your damaged blood vessels, resulting in a smaller bruise. Compressing the injury to physically stop the bleeding is even more effective. Don't try to move your ankle: using nearby muscles will attract more blood to the area which will only contribute to the developing bruise. It's harder for blood to flow uphill, so elevating your leg will also help minimise local blood flow. Conversely, if you're after an enormous bruise then apply a heat pack to your ankle and vigorously shake the affected leg while dangling it off a balcony.

Now, the part you've been waiting for – why bruises change colour. For a bruise to heal, your body must remove the trapped blood. This is done via breaking down the blood into various proteins, each of which is sequentially digested until all the blood is gone. It just so happens that each of these breakdown products is a different colour.

First up – red. Your blood is always red. Regardless of how much oxygen it's carrying, it's red. Why red? Because of red blood cells. Why are they red? Because they're full of the red protein haemoglobin (about 250 million molecules per red blood cell, to save you counting). Why is haemoglobin red? Because it contains iron, which reflects red light upon interacting with oxygen (the planet Mars, the soil in central Australia, and a rusty can are also red because of this reaction between iron and oxygen).

Not all animals transport oxygen in their blood using haemoglobin, so not all animals have red blood. Dissect a leech or segmented worm and green blood will gush out thanks to chlorocruorin, their emerald haemoglobin equivalent. Squash a marine worm and you'll create a violet puddle of hemerythrin-filled blood. Tread on a beetle or sea cucumber and you may think you've ruptured its bladder – their yellow blood is packed with the element vanadium. Some crustaceans and other arthropods use copper as their oxygen shuttle, giving their blood a blue hue. One such creature is the ironically named horseshoe crab, who is very unlucky indeed. It just so happens that their baby blue blood clots upon contact with bacteria, making it an extremely sensitive contamination detector. The sterility of vaccines, drugs and other intravenous solutions can be confirmed by the absence of clotting when mixed with horseshoe crab blood. Thousands of crabs are unwilling blood donors for the pharmaceutical industry every year. To add insult to injury humans can't even be bothered accurately naming them: they're not crabs (which are crustaceans), they're a different order of arthropods.

Haemoglobin comprises four proteins with an iron core. Those iron cores don't just account for blood's red colour, they're also why blood tastes metallic. Oxygen sticks to the iron to hitch a ride around your body. When it's carrying oxygen, haemoglobin is a vibrant red like the Coke logo. When the oxygen bails out, the haemoglobin turns a deeper beetroot red like the Dr Pepper logo. 'But wait,' you say (if you have pale skin), 'the blood in the veins at my wrist is clearly blue!' Incorrect – it just appears blue. The vein wall, plus your overlying skin and fat, absorb all light wavelengths except blue. Only blue light survives the plunge to your vein to be reflected off the deoxygenated haemoglobin and hit your eyeballs. Medieval Spanish aristocrats flaunted their pale, blue-veined skin as proof of their Gothic ancestry, uncontaminated by interbreeding with their dark-skinned Moorish enemies. This Spanish concept of *sangre azul* – blue blood – remains synonymous with royalty to this day. Your blood is always red: sometimes brighter, sometimes deeper, but always red. Don't let textbook diagrams fool you: the deoxygenated blood in your veins is as much blue as Uganda is orange in your atlas. And don't believe anyone who says that blood really is blue but turns red when you bleed because it has contacted the air. Honestly.

Put all that together and it makes sense that a fresh bruise will initially be red. Broken capillaries spew out their oxygenated, bright red blood, pooling at the site of injury. Within hours the bruise will turn bluish-purple as surrounding cells suck up any oxygen still stuck to the leaked haemoglobin. Because of skin's pernickety reflective habits, this beetroot red deoxygenated blood seen through your skin will look bluish.

Soon your body's scavengers – white blood cells – will appear on the scene. White blood cells will consume anything out of place, from bacteria to congealed bruise-blood. As they gobble up the deoxyhaemoglobin and start digesting it they produce a rainbow of products.

Given a few days your white blood cells will break down the deoxyhaemoglobin into the green compound biliverdin. A robin's eggs are turquoise due to the exact same pigment, which female robins incorporate into their eggs' shells. Healthier robins introduce more biliverdin and thus produce brighter eggs. Tiffany & Co.'s patented packaging is robin's egg blue, also known as 'Pantone 1837' after the year of Tiffany's founding. If a boastful acquaintance flaunts a Tiffany's tinted necklace, you might rein in their bragging by pointing out that its colour is shared by a bruise pigment.

Further white blood cell digestion churns biliverdin into a canary yellow product called bilirubin. Finally, any remaining iron is stored in the skin as the russet brown compound haemosiderin. Haemosiderin lingers the longest, giving old bruises their sepia hue. Post degustation, white blood cells retreat into the bloodstream and carry away with them any trace of colour. Their departure signals the final healing of your bruise.

Haemoglobin digestion happens at different rates across the bruise's surface. It may look mottled purple, yellow and green all at once. The master of mixed pigments was Vincent van Gogh, who suffered severe mental illness. Upon admission to a French psychiatric asylum in Saint-Rémy in 1889, Vincent was prescribed digitalis, a drug derived from the foxglove plant. High doses of digitalis can distort your vision by causing you to see yellow halos around objects à la *The Starry Night*. That's right: Vincent's 'yellow period' may have just been the result of a digitalis side effect rather than artistic inspiration. These days we use digitalis to treat irregular heart rhythms, but we now know that it does nothing to treat mental illness (although it could relieve anxiety if the patient was worried about their irregular heart rhythm).

As careful as you may be, you will at some point trap a fingertip in a ring binder or catch some chin flab in a bicycle helmet buckle. These hopelessly first-world problems will result in bruising. While your coordination may not impress, at least now your knowledge of the bruising process will.

SUMMARY: A bruise is trapped blood under your skin. Your body removes the blood by sequentially breaking it down into different chemicals, each of which happens to have a different colour.

AND ALSO ...

Hello, yellow

People with liver failure appear yellow – jaundiced – because the garish yellow pigment bilirubin accumulates in their skin. Their damaged livers can't break down the bilirubin that's produced by the normal turnover of red blood cells in their body. A red blood cell only lives for about 120 days. When it dies, it's broken down by white blood cells in the usual sequence: into biliverdin then bilirubin. It's your liver's job to get rid of the bilirubin now floating in your bloodstream. If your liver is healthy, it mixes the bilirubin into your bile, stores the bile in your gallbladder and eventually squirts it into your intestines. Gut bacteria convert the bilirubin into the colourless chemical urobilinogen, then break it down further into the brown-tinted stercobilin (which gives faeces their brown colour). Before it's converted into stercobilin, some of the urobilinogen seeps from your intestines back into your blood, is filtered by your kidneys and removed via your urine. When urobilinogen meets oxygen, it becomes the cheery yellow chemical urobilin, responsible for urine's buttery hue.

A damaged liver can't extract bilirubin from the blood. The built-up bilirubin, with nowhere else to go, deposits in the skin to turn it yellow. Since no bilirubin makes it through the liver into the intestines, the absence of stercobilin means the patient's faeces turn chalky white.

A foetus gets its oxygen from its mother's blood, via the placenta. But when a baby is born it needs to breathe oxygen for itself. The chemical structure of haemoglobin is different in a foetus from that in a newborn: foetal haemoglobin needs to suck oxygen from the placenta, but newborn haemoglobin needs to suck it from the air. Immediately after birth a mass turnover of red blood cells occurs as the haemoglobin switch takes place. With all the red blood cell breakdown going on, many newborns go a bit yellow: their tiny livers can't keep up with the enormous bilirubin removal burden. In severe cases the newborn's blood bilirubin levels can rise dramatically, saturate the skin and overflow into the brain. The brain literally turns bright yellow (sadly, we know this from autopsies) and permanent brain damage or death results. To prevent this awful complication, we can accelerate bilirubin breakdown by putting jaundiced newborns in what appear to be tanning beds. Blue light breaks down the bilirubin in the skin into products that the newborn's body can remove via its urine and faeces. Provision of groovy eye masks makes the treatment more enjoyable for all involved and the photos provide excellent 21st birthday party material.

Iron and grapes

Croatia's iron-laden red soil is ideal for growing grapes. Clusters of deep mauve Teran grapes are pulverised into a wine that locals vouch has the colour and taste of blood – the iron in the soil gives the wine a distinctly metallic taste.

Traditionally, Croatian women who haemorrhaged during childbirth were given Teran wine to replenish their iron stores (or just be too drunk to remember how horrific they felt).

Bruising quackery

Some ancient cultures (and some modern quacks) deliberately inflicted bruises to 'treat' various ailments. Called cupping, the technique involves placing hollow devices over the skin and producing suction via cooling or pumps. The pressure ruptures underlying capillaries and causes an impressive bruise. It was claimed that this sucked out various loosely-defined 'toxins' from the body. A Neo-Assyrian clay tablet dating from 700 BC describes 'cupping by sucking, with the mouth or by using a buffalo horn'. Incidentally, a hickey, or love bite, is a bruise formed by sucking with the mouth, performed for non-medicinal purposes.

A bruise you really don't want

A hairline fracture is not a fracture of your hairline, but a tiny hair-like crack in a bone. However, fractures of your hairline are indeed possible. Skull fractures can be particularly nasty, given the numerous important soft organs nearby that function best when not impaled by bone shards. Certain tell-tale bruises around the eyes ('raccoon eyes') and ears suggest that the base of the skull at the nape of the neck has been fractured. The bruises behind the ears are called 'Battle's sign', after surgeon William Henry Battle who first described them in *The Lancet* in 1890 alongside some sensible advice:

> ... unless search is made for the extravasation, [Battle's sign] is very apt to be overlooked, as the ear conceals it, especially if the ear is large or the head of the patient has not been shaved.[3]

ENDNOTES

1   World Population Prospects 2019: Ten Key Findings. *United Nations, Department of Economic and Social Affairs, Population Division* (2019).

2   Malarchuk, C. & Dan Robson, D. *A Matter of Inches*. Triumph Books (2014).

3   Battle, W. H. Lectures on some points relating to injuries to the head. *Lancet*, 1, 57–63 (1890).

ITCH

'Happiness is having a scratch for every itch.'
Ogdon Nash

Being unable to relieve an itch is intensely frustrating. NASA astronauts stick squares of Velcro inside their helmets within reach of their nose in case they need to scratch during a spacewalk. According to Apollo 17 astronaut Harrison Schmitt, 'Everybody seemed to agree that you needed that [bit of Velcro]'. Self-inflicted itch as a form of penitence dates back to the Old Testament. Pious preachers wore itchy undershirts against their skin, usually made from rough sackcloth or coarse woven animal hair, to mortify their flesh and atone for their sins. Lice often infested the shirts, further intensifying the itch. The medieval emperor Charlemagne was buried in a hairshirt. Thomas Beckett, the Archbishop of Canterbury, was wearing one when disgruntled noblemen hacked him to death in Canterbury Cathedral in 1170. Sir Thomas More sported a hairshirt while he was imprisoned in the Tower of London in 1529.

In Molière's 1669 comedy *Tartuffe* ('The Hypocrite'), the title character commands his servant to 'hang up my hair shirt'. The hypocrite's hypocrisy is threefold: 1) wearing a hairshirt was usually a private act between the wearer and God, 2) a repentant Christian shouldn't really be ordering around a servant, and 3) taking off a hairshirt defeats its purpose. Itch didn't just torment hairshirt-wearing Christians on Earth: an eternity of itch might await them in the afterlife. In Dante's 14th century poem Inferno (Italian for 'Hell'), the perpetual punishment awaiting falsifiers was 'the burning rage of fierce itching which nothing could relieve'.

If itch is hell, and war is hell, then being itchy in the trenches must be as infernal as it gets. Relentless itch tormented men on the frontline in World War I. Body lice swarmed over the soldiers whose skin became riddled with bites. Containing the infestation was impossible in the crowded conditions. The soldiers' skin and uniforms became caked in lice and the insects' faeces. Routine appointments at 'delousing stations' to douse louse-filled uniforms in naphthalene (the main chemical in mothballs) achieved little, besides making the men smell like their grandparents' cupboards, which may have at least been nostalgically comforting. Vigorous washing dislodged the lice, but their sticky eggs persisted. Mere hours after donning freshly laundered clothes, the men's body heat had incubated the hidden eggs to hatching point, releasing yet another generation of lice. Deranged by itch, soldiers would hold flames to their bodies to incinerate the critters, relishing the satisfying 'crack' as the lice exploded. Isaac Rosenberg, a soldier and one of England's most celebrated trench poets during World War I, captured the maddening itch in his poem *The Immortals* (1918):

> I killed them, but they would not die.
> Yea! all the day and all the night
> For them I could not rest or sleep,
> Nor guard from them nor hide in flight.
> Then in my agony I turned
> And made my hands red in their gore.
> In vain – for faster than I slew
> They rose more cruel than before.
> I killed and killed with slaughter mad;
> I killed till all my strength was gone.
> And still they rose to torture me,

For Devils only die in fun.
I used to think the Devil hid
In women's smiles and wine's carouse.
I called him Satan, Balzebub;
But now I call him, dirty louse.[1]

Alas, those dirty, immortal lice were even more devilish than Rosenberg knew. Itchy bites were just the beginning: the body lice also spread disease via their faeces. Every time a louse defecated it deposited bacteria on the soldier's skin. If a soldier squashed (or thermally 'cracked') a louse, its bacteria-laden entrails would splatter over his body. Vigorous scratching, often drawing blood, rubbed these bacteria into his bite wounds and created further skin breaks which soon became infected. Two louse-borne bacteria produced epidemics in World War I. *Bartonella quintana* caused trench fever, a relatively mild illness typified by fever and shin pain. But the other bacterium, *Rickettsia prowazekii*, was responsible for a far typhus deadlier disease. Typhus is from the Greek for 'hazy', a reference to the profoundly confused mental state of those affected, who also suffer fever, rash, muscle pain and a plummeting blood pressure. Typhus epidemics decimated the Eastern Front with some 30 million cases and three million deaths. Lenin knew that lice were making his men drop like flies. At the Seventh All-Russian Congress of Soviets, in December 1919, he announced: 'We must concentrate everything on this problem. Either the lice will defeat socialism, or socialism will defeat the lice!'

*

In 1600, German physician Samuel Hafenreffer offered a roundabout definition of itch: '… an unpleasant sensation that elicits the desire or reflex to scratch.' It's an accurate description of the familiar chain of events, but not very useful for the reader seeking to understand how itch actually works. (Rather reminiscent of lexicographer Samuel Johnson's definition of 'lizard' in his 1755 *Dictionary of the English Language*: 'something resembling a serpent, with legs added to it.') In the 400-odd years since Hafenreffer's stab at defining itch, we've sent men to the moon and invented spray-on cheese. But we still haven't worked out how itch works.

Let's start with what we *do* know. The sensation of itch draws your attention to skin irritants. Your skin is the first line of defence against infection: the barrier between your internal organs and the germ-ridden outside world. Broken skin is about as useful as an armoured car with its windows wound down. Feeling itchy drives you to scratch, an action that dislodges potential skin-harmers before they sting, pierce, contaminate or otherwise sully your surface. Itch/scratch behaviour is a widely used infection prevention technique across the animal kingdom. Seals scrub their heads with flippers, horses scrape their mangy manes against fence posts, worm-infested dogs drag their itching anuses across the carpet, and even fruit flies rub themselves if they have a mite infection (yes, flies can get mites; bacteria can get viruses too).

Your ability to dislodge biting insects before they can puncture your skin relies on the sensation of itch induced by their scampering feet. Their filthy mouthparts can directly contaminate your bloodstream with the bugs responsible for malaria, dengue fever, yellow fever, Zika virus, Japanese encephalitis and Lyme disease – just to name a few. But it's not only biting insects that can transmit disease. Disturbing research in 2017[2] revealed that house flies harbour more than 300 types of bacteria, from *E. coli* to *Helicobacter pylori* (the bug behind stomach ulcers). The wings and feet of the flies were found to be particularly heavily infested, 'suggesting that bacteria use the flies as airborne shuttles', as researcher Stephan Schuster put it.

*

Consider the remarkable range of sensations that your skin can discriminate between. The light brush of a cat's tail; the pressure of a lumpy mattress digging into your back; the vibration of an electric toothbrush against your palm; the itch of a rough woollen sleeve; the pain of a poorly deployed staple. Your skin is so touchy because it's jam-packed with sensory receptors. Think of them as tiny antennae, each wired up to your central nervous system via nerves in your peripheries. Anything that touches your skin triggers some of these sensory receptors, causing them to fire off a message that travels along those nerves to let your brain know about it.

Certain parts of your body need to have more sensitive skin than others: your fingertips for manual dexterity and finding the end of a roll of sticky-tape; your genitals to protect your genetic line (if just a gentle knock causes eye-watering pain, you'll soon learn to protect your baby-making machinery. Plus, pleasant sensations during copulation encourage you to breed). Conversely, having a super-sensitive upper back capable of reading Braille, for example, is not particularly useful. The sensitivity of any particular patch of skin depends on how densely packed it is with sensory receptors. The skin on your calf only has a smattering of sensory receptors. Conversely, your exquisitely sensitive fingertips are brimming with sensory receptors that will perceive even the slightest stimulation.

Each of the sensations that your skin can detect has its own specially shaped, exotically named receptor type. That's why you don't confuse your phone buzzing in your pocket with a bee sting: different skin sensations (like vibration and pain) trigger different sensory receptors. Let me introduce you to them. 'Meissner's corpuscle' are your skin's sausage-shaped sensory receptors that detect light touch.* Pressure activates the candelabra-like

---

* Georg Meissner (1829–1905), a German anatomist who studied medicine in *Göttingen* (a town famous for its sausages, as it happens)

projections of your skin's 'Merkel's discs'.* Vibrations set your skin's 'Pacinian corpuscles'† trembling (they look uncannily like onions). Football-shaped 'Ruffini endings'‡ are the sensory receptors that detect skin stretch.

When it comes to detecting the unpleasant sensations of itch and pain, your skin economically uses a shared sensory receptor. Unlike the other receptors, it doesn't have a creative shape or a weird name. The antennae that detect itch and pain look like frayed ropes and are called nociceptors, from the Latin for 'to harm' (*nocere*). Nociceptors keep your brain in the loop about potentially harmful stimuli touching your skin.

Isn't it curious that the same sensory receptors – nociceptors – respond to both itch and pain? It suggests that these sensations are related. You're right. But the nature of the relationship is complicated.

Researchers used to think of itch as just a milder form of pain. The two sensations represented opposite ends of the unpleasant skin sensation spectrum, detected by the same receptors and travelling along the same nerve pathways to your brain. A mild irritant (like a hairshirt against your skin) caused itch; a major irritant (like stepping barefoot on a wayward piece of Lego) caused pain. But you might have already identified some problems with this intensity theory. The pain from treading on Lego doesn't dissipate into an itch. If you step lightly on Lego, it doesn't itch, it just hurts a bit less. A fresh mosquito bite becomes increasingly itchy, but never feels painful. Plus, your reactions to itch and pain are poles apart. Your response to itch is to confront the irritant

---

* Friedrich Sigmund Merkel (1845-1919), a German anatomist who introduced the 'red for arteries, blue for veins' colour-coding system for medical texts that has misled people about blood's true colour ever since (see *Bruising*, page 244).

† Filippo Pacini (1812-1883), an Italian anatomist credited with isolating *Vibrio cholerae*, the bacterium behind cholera.

‡ Angelo Ruffini (1864-1929), an Italian anatomist with an interest in amphibian embryos.

with a scratch; your response to pain is to yank the affected body part away.

But pause for a moment and think about what scratching actually is: it's self-inflicted pain. Vigorously scratch the back of your hand and you'll agree that in the absence of itch, scratching hurts. If you've got an itch, however, scratching isn't painful: it's paradise. Itchy skin can be alleviated by other sources of mild pain besides scratching, like ice and capsaicin (the chemical that makes chillies hot).

Why should pain relieve itch? It's a quirk of how your nociceptors work: when they're confronted with both itchy and painful stimuli, they put the itch signal on hold and prioritise pain.

Fair enough: a flesh wound warrants attention sooner than an itchy elbow. Scratching an itch feels heavenly because the slight pain you're causing makes your brain releases the mood-enhancing neurotransmitter serotonin. But the bliss is short-lived. That same serotonin amplifies the itch signals travelling up your spinal cord. Before long, your itch will return with a vengeance. It takes serious willpower to break the itch/scratch vicious circle, as those of us who've scraped away at a mosquito bite until it bled know all too well.

The current thinking is that pain and itch are distinct sensations. But itch researchers remain split into two camps when it comes to how we sense an itch. The 'specificity theory' punters think that some nociceptors only respond to itch, not pain as well, and that these itch messages travel along itch-specific nerves to the brain. Conversely, the 'pattern theory' crew reckon that all the sensors and cabling for nociception are identical, but differences in firing patterns allow your brain to distinguish between irritants that itch and irritants that hurt.

When it comes to itch research, we've only scratched the surface.

*

If you're feeling itchy, the itch initiator can usually be narrowed down to one of three suspects: your skin, an itch-inducing chemical, or your brain.

Skin-based itch

Dry skin, like a dry riverbed, forms cracks. It's prone to itch because irritants can slip down those fissures to directly trigger your nociceptors. Skin becomes dehydrated if it loses its usual waterproof layer of sebum (see *Acne*, page 278). Common sebum-strippers include overzealous washing, aging, sunburn and low humidity, air-conditioned environments. People with eczema (also called atopic dermatitis, because nobody can spell eczema) struggle to maintain moist skin due to a faulty skin barrier that's prone to inflammation. Inherited defects in the gene for filaggrin, the protein glue that holds your skin cells together, are often to blame. Like a brick wall with crumbling mortar, faulty filaggrin results in cracked, sensitive skin. Heavy-duty moisturisers are the backbone of eczema treatment.

Children with eczema struggle to understand the importance of not scratching. Desperate parents are taught to clip their child's fingernails short and tape cotton gloves to their hands overnight. But the urge to scratch is so strong that children often cover themselves in bleeding, infected scratch wounds. I once worked in a paediatric eczema clinic where my job was to slather children with moisturiser, then bandage their limbs from end to end to give the cream a chance to seep in. The poor kids had to keep the bandages on for as long as possible, while enduring relentless taunting from unsympathetic siblings. To make the process less traumatic, I encouraged the children to pretend they were mummified zombies, committing to the role by chasing their siblings, bandaged arms outstretched, while emitting a low moan. I heard that this was a particularly effective anti-teasing technique.

Chemical-based itch

If certain chemicals contact your skin – like those in poison ivy, insect spit, chickenpox blisters, things you're allergic to, and novelty itching powders – your skin responds by releasing itch-inducing substances that send your nociceptors into overdrive. Histamine is the most potent of these chemicals. A nociceptor, when doused in histamine, sends your brain such a powerful itch signal that it can induce self-mutilation. Many adults harbour pock-marked faces: scars from picking at histamine-laden chickenpox spots as a child.

Histamine is responsible for the infuriating itch of a mosquito bite. A mosquito begins its meal by piercing your skin with its straw-like proboscises (yes, plural: their mouth javelin comprises six small spears, not one) Before it starts sucking up your blood, it dribbles some saliva into you. As expected, your skin responds to chemicals in the mosquito saliva by releasing a flood of histamine. So why is the itch delayed? Those cursed mosquitoes have developed a cunning adaptation to evade our scratch defence: their spit contains a local anaesthetic which renders you oblivious to the mosquito's presence. By the time the numbness wears off the bloated mosquito has flown far away. The unmasked itch is so intense because that mosquito didn't just spit into you once: it was constantly regurgitating while it was feeding. Mosquitos only want to fill up on your red blood cells, not the watery plasma that those cells float in. To conserve stomach space, the mosquito spews your plasma back into you, infusing your skin with more saliva which triggers even more histamine release – and one hell of an itch.

Itch-inducing chemicals don't always come from your environment: they can also be internally generated by failing organs. Your kidneys and liver are responsible for cleansing your blood of the junk by-products dumped there by your body's constant chemical reactions. If either organ isn't working, itch can result as the waste chemicals accumulate in your blood, leach into your skin and set off your nociceptors. Urea is the chemical culprit in kidney failure. The skin can become so saturated that urea oozes from the pores, crystallising on the skin to leave an icing sugar-like coating called 'uraemic frost'. The Greek physician Aretaeus first described liver failure-related itch over 2000 years ago, blaming the symptom on 'prickly bilious particles'. Peculiarly, patients with liver failure tend to have particularly strong itch on their palms and soles of their feet.

Brain-driven itch

Ultimately, it's your brain that decides if you're itchy. Nociceptors in your skin can send your brain all the itch messages they want, but it's your brain's job to interpret those signals and determine an appropriate response. Multiple brain areas are activated by an incoming itch message, including regions for emotional processing (reflecting the unpleasantness of feeling itchy) and impulse control (namely, the overwhelming desire to scratch). Your mood also affects how itchy you feel. In a 2012 study published in *The British Journal of Dermatology*, subjects felt itchier after watching film clips from an 'emotionally negative' movie (*Irreversible*, in which a man seeks revenge on his girlfriend's rapist) than after viewing positive film clips (from *Happy Feet*, in which penguins tap dance and sing).[3]

As the final arbiter, it follows that your brain can produce the sensation of itch all by itself. Brain-generated itch is particularly distressing. Since there's no itchy irritant to remove from the skin, scratching provides no relief: it's like trying to correct a typo by slathering white-out on your computer screen.

Delusional parasitosis is a psychiatric disorder where the patient holds the fixed false belief that they're infested with bugs of some description. Sufferers often experience 'formication' (not to be confused with fornication) – the sensation of insects crawling on the skin – from the Latin *formica*, meaning 'ant'. I once treated a chef who presented with extensive skin burns, not from a kitchen mishap, but due to the daily undiluted bleach baths he'd been taking to kill the non-existent bugs he believed were crawling over him. Treatment with antipsychotic medication allowed him to return to a normal life. Methamphetamines like ice and speed can produce vivid visual hallucinations of skin-scampering insects accompanied by intense formication. Apparently, users refer to these imaginary bugs as 'meth mites', 'crank bugs' and, my personal favourite, 'amphetamites' (I received this etymology/entomology lesson from an ice user who had attended the emergency department with infected scratch wounds).

This chapter has probably made you itchy. I've certainly been regularly scratching while writing it. When your attention is drawn to itch, your impressionable brain encourages you to join in. Itch is a contagious behaviour, like yawning (see *Yawning*, page 54). But while contagious yawning abounds among highly empathetic people, the same can't be said for contagious itch. A 2012 paper titled 'Neural basis of contagious itch and why some people are more prone to it' found that empathy was irrelevant as a predictor for susceptibility to contagious itch; instead, it was the more neurotic people – those who tended to experience more negative emotions – who were predisposed to catching an itch.[4] What's more, contagious yawning is restricted to socially advanced primates, but even dumb mice (no offence, mice) can catch an itch. Contagious itch probably evolved as a way to contain parasitic infestations. Increased scratching among fellow tribespeople may herald a lice outbreak. By joining in, you could dislodge any lice that might have already scuttled from your neighbour onto you.

That's how lice spread between humans: by physical contact. Nit-removal clinics have reported surges in business around the time that *Pixar* movies are released owing to lice springing from child to child in crowded cinemas. Humans host a triad of distinct lice species: head, pubic and body lice. Head lice prefer the thinner hair on our head; pubic lice seek the thicker locks of our armpits, genitals, eyelashes and beards; while body lice live in your clothes until they feel hungry.

'Nits' refer to head lice eggs, not the critters themselves. 'Crabs' is slang for pubic lice because these critters look uncannily like crabs, claws included. The Greek for crab is *cancer*, hence the crab-shaped constellation's name and associated star-sign. Cancer – the disease – was named by doctors who thought that the swollen veins radiating from tumours were reminiscent of a crab. British soldiers referred to body lice as 'cooties', a slang term that has evolved to cover the full spectrum of lice – body, head and pubic. Entomologists asked etymologists to explain this term, who suggested that it may come from the Malay term for lice, *kutu*. But since most British soldiers didn't speak Malay, a more likely origin story is that 'cooties' is derived from the coot, a type of waterfowl regarded as particularly parasite-ridden.

SUMMARY: Itch is an unpleasant skin sensation that makes you want to scratch. Itch protects your skin from irritants like insects that might breach your skin and cause infection.

AND ALSO …

On whales and barnacle penises

Breaching whales are a majestic sight, but why do they do it? The majestic leaps might communicate physical fitness to other whales, or just be playful fun. Or perhaps they breach for another reason: because they're itchy. Stumpy whale flippers can't reach very far to scratch off the swarms of parasites scurrying over their skin. But when a whale flings its gargantuan body skyward and smashes back onto the water, it sends those critters flying. Whales must particularly loathe the male barnacles glued to their surface whose tentacle-like penises (eight times their body length, the longest penis relative to body size of any animal) probably tickle their host as they rove relentlessly over the whale's skin in search of a female barnacle's orifice. Alas, what holidaymakers are really paying for on a whale-watching tour is the opportunity to observe an irritated humpback repeatedly trying to dislodge humping barnacles from its back.

Tracking down the spinal tract for itch

Itch and pain signals travel along the same nerve bundles in your spinal cord. Doctors discovered this fact due to an unexpected side-effect of a spinal cord operation called a cordotomy. The procedure was devised in 1912 as a last-ditch treatment for patients with severe pain on one side of their body, like a tumour eroding a leg bone. At the time, it was known that pain messages reached your brain via bundles of nerves on either side of your spinal cord. Like snipping a telephone wire, surgically slicing through one of those bundles would block pain messages from half the body (the half with the painful leg tumour, for example) from getting to the patient's brain.

Operating just below the patient's earlobe, the surgeon performing the cordotomy would cut through the skin, fat, muscle and bone until the spinal cord was on show. After taking a deep breath (I assume), the surgeon would then slice a few millimetres through the side of the spinal cord to sever the pain-carrying tract on that side. Post-op, the patient would be unable to feel pain down one half of their body as planned. But curiously, patients noticed that the same half also became completely insensitive to itch. Case reports soon dotted the medical literature. One cordotomy patient was oblivious to poison ivy rubbed on his painless side. The authors of a 1950 article published in the journal *Brain* noted that their cordotomy patients were not 'annoyed by the itch' of mosquito bites.[5] The conclusion was clear: the pain-carrying nerve bundle that the surgeons cut during a cordotomy must also carry itch messages. Incidentally, Sir Henry Head was *Brain*'s head editor from 1905 to 1923. Ridiculously, in 1954, Sir Russell Brain became the head of *Brain*. Sir Brain also authored a number of confusingly titled neurology texts including 'Brain's Diseases of the Nervous System' and 'Brain's Clinical Neurology'.

ENDNOTES

1   Rosenberg, I. The Immortals. The Isaac Rosenberg Literary Estate, The Imperial War Museum. *First World War Poetry Digital Archive.* http://ww1lit. nsms.ox.ac.uk/ww1lit/collections/document/1703.

2   Junqueira, A. C. M. et al. The Microbiomes of Blowflies and Houseflies as Bacterial Transmission Reservoirs. *Scientific Reports*, 7 (1) (2017).

3   Laarhoven, A. I. M. et al. Role of Induced Negative and Positive Emotions in Sensitivity to Itch and Pain in Women. *British Journal of Dermatology*, 167 (2), 262–69 (2012).

4   Holle, H. et al. Neural basis of contagious itch and why some people are more prone to it. *Proceedings of the National Academy of Sciences*, 109 (48), 19816–19821 (2012).

5   White J. C, et al. Anterolateral cordotomy: Results, complications and causes of failure. *Brain*, 73, 346–67 (1950).

ALLERGIES

What has a shell, is energy-dense and kills thousands of people every year? Improvised explosive devices ... and peanuts.

I once treated an American teenager who told me that he was allergic to Vegemite (he said it made him nauseated) and eucalyptus (scented toilet spray made his eyes water). He was mistaken; taste and smell aversions are not allergies. Instead, this lad's reported 'allergies' were probably a redirection of resentment towards his father (who had relocated the family to Melbourne for work) manifesting as a dislike of Australian food and flora. Usually I would have jumped at the chance to explain how allergies actually worked. But he was partially anaesthetised and about to have an abscess on his left buttock excised, so I figured this was not the time.

An allergy is not the generic term for any negative outcome following exposure to something. Many so-called allergies are just side-effects. For example, you're not 'allergic' to opioid painkillers like codeine and fentanyl if they make you constipated. As well as blocking pain receptors, opioids decrease your intestinal squeezing rate, meaning faeces stay in your body longer. You're not 'allergic' to aspirin and similar drugs like ibuprofen if they make your stomach hurt. These drugs restrict your stomach's ability to ooze out mucous, rendering its uncoated walls prone to acid erosion and ulcers. For a bad reaction to be an allergy, the damage must be caused by your immune system.

The immune system refers to the cells, chemicals and tissues that help your body fend off infection. It performs constant surveillance for foreign invaders like bacteria and viruses. The guards are white blood cells (they're actually transparent, not white: the name comes from the fact they lack the scarlet pigment of red blood cells). They bob up in your blood, loiter in your skin and coat your gut and airways. White blood cells scrutinise everything you touch, inhale and eat. From their point of view, your body contains things that should be there (such as kidneys), can be there (like ingested asparagus), and shouldn't be there (pinworms, for instance). A well-behaved immune system ignores the kidneys, tolerates the asparagus but seeks to destroy anything in that third category.

Problems arise when the immune system gets the categorisation wrong. We want it to attack pinworms and other members of the shouldn't-be-there category – like bacteria, viruses, and fungi – since this keeps us healthy; but when the immune system attacks things in the other two categories, it is decidedly unhelpful. Attacks on things that should be there cause autoimmune diseases: a pancreas attack results in type 1 diabetes, for example, while joint attacks occur in rheumatoid arthritis. Attacks on things that can be there (like pollen and latex gloves) result in allergies.

We don't know exactly why some people have allergies. Consider identical twins, who have identical DNA. If one twin has a peanut allergy, there's only a 64 per cent chance that the other twin will share the allergy. Clearly, allergies aren't purely genetic: there must be some environmental influence too. If the environment is right (well, wrong, actually) and you've got the genetic predisposition: you might just develop an allergy.

Let's start with the environmental factors. The air you breathe, the range of food you've swallowed, the breeds of bacteria you've been exposed to (touched, eaten, drunk, inhaled, rubbed in your eyes): these all affect your chances of developing an allergy. The 'hygiene hypothesis' proposes that inadequate exposure to allergy-causing substances as a child increases the risk of developing an allergy. Since your immune system hasn't 'encountered' a wide range of potential invaders and thus learnt that the majority are safe, it reacts excessively when exposed to harmless substances. Consider hay fever. In 1873, English physician Charles Blakely opined:

> Hay fever is said to be an aristocratic disease, and there
> can be no doubt that, if it is not almost wholly confined to
> the upper classes of society, it is rarely, if ever met with but
> among the educated.[1]

Blakely was slightly invested in this flattering description: he himself had hay fever. He claimed that all his patients with pollen allergy were refined men like him: doctors, clergymen or military men. Blakely's suggested cures were equally upper class: a 'sojourn at the seaside' or a 'cruise in a yacht'. Those 'cures' worked because they removed the sufferer from flora-heavy habitats; being locked in a cupboard would also be an effective hay fever cure.

As it happens, hay fever doesn't have a mysterious predilection for toffs. Instead, Blakely's observations can be explained by the hygiene hypothesis. Aristocrats likely spent a sheltered childhood indoors, occupied with Latin lessons and playing pranks on their butler. Children born into lower class farming families, however, were harvesting rye before they had teeth. Ample pollen exposure in their early life taught their immune system that pollen was safe. But that posh kid might first encounter rye grass pollen, say, on a tour of his diocese as an adult. Not having encountered this substance before, his immune system would attack the pollen, just as it would attack any other unrecognised invader like influenza viruses. The result? A holy hay fever trinity of swollen eyes, runny nose and scratchy throat.

Let's now consider the genetic factors that make people prone to allergies. As usual, Charles Darwin can help us explain how a genetic propensity to allergies may have evolved: the survival of the fittest. Early humans with lazy immune systems that overlooked *Salmonella* bacteria say, would die from infection before they could pass on their genes. Those equipped with more sensitive immune systems that could recognise *Salmonella* would survive, passing on their 'sensitive immune system' genes to their offspring. As the generations continued, natural selection of these fitter humans resulted in increasing immune system sensitivity. But increased sensitivity is only beneficial to a point when it comes to immune systems. Eventually this process produced humans whose immune systems were too sensitive: ones that overreacted to harmless substances like pollen and peanuts – that is, they suffered allergies.

People with oversensitive immune systems haven't died out because most allergic reactions aren't deadly. So long as their intermittently puffy eyes and streaming noses don't deter all potential partners, they can still breed and pass on their genes. From an evolutionary standpoint, it's better to have a twitchy, allergic reaction-causing immune system than a sluggish one. Mistakenly attacking pollen might cause itchy hives but it won't end your genetic line like overlooking measles will. Through evolution, we've ended up as a species equipped with immune systems that usually get the balance right but are sometimes too sensitive and result in allergies.

None of these explanations fully explains everything about allergies. Like why an adult might suddenly develop a dog allergy after decades of owning a dachshund. Or why some people outgrow their allergies. Or why the universe would be so cruel as to give Buddy Ebsen, the actor originally cast as the Tin Man in the 1939 production of *The Wizard of Oz*, an allergy to the aluminium dust used in the makeup, forcing him to resign and spend a fortnight in hospital with respiratory failure. Or why some people seem drawn to work with the thing they're allergic to, like Brian Radam (curator of the British Lawnmower museum; allergic to grass) or Ian Wragg (children's magician in County Durham, England; forced to retire due to an allergy to the rabbits he pulled from his hat). Sometimes it seems like the immune system, too, works via magic.

*

Just like the immune systems of their patients, immunologists are super-sensitive when it comes to allergy terminology. To avoid upsetting them, let's clarify some definitions before we go any further. The thing that you're allergic to is called an 'allergen' (it's *allergy-gen*erating). The specific chemical chunk of that allergen that sets off your immune system is called an 'antigen' (*anti*body *gen*erating). The Y-shaped protein that your immune system makes in response to that antigen is the 'antibody' (*anti*-toxin *body*). The Y-shape is useful: two arms to seize the antigen, plus a handy stem that other immune cells can grab on to. Adopt a stance with your arms in the air to make a 'Y' to simulate an antibody. Your hands represent the variable part: both identical, and both precisely shaped to grasp onto a specific antigen – part of a peanut's chemical structure, for example.

Say you're allergic to eggs. The first time you ate an omelette you wouldn't have noticed anything. Unbeknownst to you, your immune system detected the egg antigens in your body and erroneously categorised them as 'shouldn't be there' instead of 'can be there'. Panicking, your immune system began churning out egg-specific antibodies: ones whose Y 'hands' specifically docked onto egg antigens. This process – the first time your immune system freaked out at that harmless egg antigen and made antibodies – is called sensitisation. These anti-egg antibodies dispersed body wide. They embedded their Y-trunks into white blood cells called mast cells, leaving their egg-seeking hands pointing outwards, poised to snatch any egg antigens that might pass by in the future. The name 'mast cell' comes from the German *Mastzellen* ('fattened' or 'well-fed' cell) because these lardy cells are bloated with the chemical histamine – the source of your allergy symptoms.

In the event of a second eggsperience, swallowed egg antigens soon bump into those egg-seeking antibody hands poking out from your mast cells. The chemical binding of antigen to antibody – egg protein to Y-hand – triggers the underlying mast cell to splatter its histamine entrails into the surrounding tissue. The general effect of the histamine spray is to expand everything in its path. Histamine-splashed blood vessels widen. Extra blood flow brings more white blood cells to join the egg attack. The histamine-doused area – for example your lips and tongue – swells from the extra fluid. The itch is due to histamine activating nearby nerve fibres. Taking an antihistamine tablet, as the name suggests, can alleviate your symptoms by neutralising the excess histamine.

Your specific allergy symptoms depend on the location of allergen contact and subsequent deluge of histamine. Touching, inhaling or eating the allergen will result in a puffy hand, trachea or tongue respectively. What if the location of allergen contact is your genitalia? This was the focus of an engrossing 2007 case report: 'Dangerous Liaison: sexually transmitted allergic reaction to Brazil nuts'.[2] The 20-year-old woman in question, 'shortly after vaginal intercourse with her partner', developed widespread hives and 'suffered significant itching and swelling of her vagina'. Her thoughtful partner had been very careful:

> ... [he] was aware of the patient's very significant nut allergy and had bathed, brushed his teeth and cleaned his nails immediately before intercourse as he had consumed mixed nuts roughly two to three hours earlier. These had included between four to five Brazil nuts.

Doctors hypothesised that perhaps her partner's semen had contained traces of Brazil nuts. If a man eats Brazil nuts, do Brazil nut proteins (antigens) gravitate towards his anatomical nuts and become incorporated into his semen? To test this idea, they asked the man for two semen samples: one before eating

Brazil nuts, then another a few hours after munching on a handful of Brazils. Doctors dripped these samples on her skin, 'with the patient's consent' (thank goodness). The first sample: no skin reaction. The post-Brazil sample? A large hive erupted. 'We believe this to be the first case of a sexually transmitted allergic reaction,' the authors concluded, but 'unfortunately the couple separated soon afterwards, and it was impossible to formally confirm the secretion of Brazil nut proteins into seminal fluid by ... other techniques'. Her allergic reaction in this scenario could have been prevented by the use of a condom, unless she was allergic to latex too.

On condoms, a 'prophylactic' is a euphemism for a condom, from the Greek for 'protection'. The opposite of prophylaxis, then, is anaphylaxis ('against protection'). Rather than protect the body, an immune system in anaphylactic shock fails like a perforated prophylactic. Anaphylaxis is the severest form of allergy. Uncontrolled floodgates of histamine and other inflammatory chemicals open en masse throughout the body, not just localised to where you contacted the allergen. Your blood pressure plummets from profound blood vessel dilation. Blood-deprived organs start to fail. Fluid seeps from leaky blood vessels into the surrounding tissues: your eyelids swell shut and your swollen tongue plugs your trachea. Even if you could shove it past your engorged tongue, an antihistamine tablet would be woefully inadequate in this situation. Your only hope of survival is high-dose adrenaline, immediately. Nothing else works. Adrenaline, a hormone naturally produced by your adrenal glands, counteracts histamine. It tightens blood vessels, melts away tissue swelling, and opens up the airways. Without adrenaline, anaphylaxis can kill within 15 minutes. Even with adrenaline, severe anaphylaxis can be unstoppable.

EpiPens (named after the American term for adrenaline, 'epinephrine' in a pen-shaped device) are brightly bi-coloured portable adrenaline needles that everyone with a serious allergy should have on hand. In the event of an allergic reaction, shove the orange end of the pen hard against the side of your thigh (don't worry about dropping your jeans first: the needle is sharp) and press the blue end to deploy the needle. The rhyme 'blue to the sky, orange to the thigh' reminds users, whose eyelids may be rapidly swelling shut, that the orange end of the EpiPen is the pointy bit and the blue end is the 'press here to inject adrenaline' bit. Accidentally flipping the EpiPen the other way and injecting adrenaline into your thumb can cause the local blood vessels to tighten so much that your thumb loses blood supply, shrivels up, and dies. Although you may have already died from anaphylaxis first.

The term anaphylaxis was coined in 1902 by French physiologist Charles Richet. While on a cruise on a yacht (during an oceanography expedition; he wasn't following Dr Blakely's hay fever treatment advice), Richet injected dogs with the venom from the tentacles of some sea anemones and Portuguese men o' war. No reaction. Twenty-two days later he injected the dogs again. The dogs became incredibly unwell and died 25 minutes later. That first injection had sensitised the pooches; the second had triggered anaphylaxis. His research didn't win friends among animal rights activists, but it did win him the 1913 Nobel Prize for Physiology or Medicine. In his acceptance speech, Richet concluded:

> Anaphylaxis, perhaps a sorry matter for the individual, is necessary to the species, often to the detriment of the individual. The individual may perish, it does not matter. The species must at any time keep its organic integrity intact.

SUMMARY: Allergies happen when your immune system overreacts to something harmless. They are the price humans pay for having an immune system that can detect and eliminate truly dangerous invaders. Some unfortunate people happen to have an immune system that's a bit loose on the 'invader' definition.

AND ALSO ...

Remember immune memory when you get your next vaccine

I'm allergic to bees, so it's easy for me to remember that the immune cells that generate antibodies are called 'B cells'.* Whether the invader is bee venom or tetanus toxin, it's B cells that make the antibodies to combat it. During an infection, antibodies have two main purposes. First, when a swarm of antibodies clings paparazzi-style to a pathogen, they physically thwart its spread. Second, your immune system's microbe-munching white blood cells view anything tagged by antibodies as 'awaiting destruction'.

Say you're infected with measles for the first time. Your B cells will take about four days to recognise the infection and start cranking out measles-specific antibodies. Antibody production will peak on about day 10 then drop off as the infection clears. But B cells are only slow the first time. If they encounter measles again, 'memory B cells' lingering from the first infection will start pumping out measles-specific antibodies within a day. The encore is also longer and stronger: the activated memory B cells can churn out 100 to 1000 times more antibodies than during the debut response.

What if we could skip that first slow, clumsy B cell dress rehearsal? That first measles infection would have been much less severe if you already had measles-specific memory B cells waiting in the wings who were familiar with the war plan. It turns out you *can* skip the dress rehearsal: by getting a vaccine.

---

* Your B cells are made in your bone marrow, but the B doesn't stand for 'bone'. Instead, the 'B' is for the 'Bursa of Fabricius', the site of B cell production in birds. Italian anatomist Hieronymus Fabricius first identified the bursa in 1621, located in the bird's cloaca (their multipurpose single orifice for urination, defecation, and copulation).

Most vaccines contain a sample of a pathogen that can't make you sick but gives your immune system a sneak peek at the bug's molecular appearance – an antigen like the microbe's outer casing, or a particular chemical chunk of it. In the days after your vaccine injection, that slow debut B cell response occurs. Your B cells recognise the injected antigen as foreign, spew out a few antibodies whose hands specifically grab the injected antigen, then form memory B cells. Dress rehearsal complete. If you're ever infected with real tetanus/measles/mumps, those memory B cells will immediately wake up. Bug-specific antibodies will surge forth in one day instead of four and the invasion will be rapidly contained, ideally so fast that you don't even fall ill.

Thyme for the thymus

During childhood, your immune system learns to recognise the cells that make up your own body – like your pancreatic and kidney cells – and appropriately ignores them. The schooling takes place in the thymus gland, a thyme leaf-shaped gland that sits just behind the top of your breastbone. Within your thymus, newborn white blood cells called 'T cells' (T stands for thymus) get challenged with various examples of 'self'. A sample of your skin cells perhaps, or a taster of your testicular tissue. If the baby T cell violently launches an attack on these self-samples, that T cell is instantly destroyed. Only self-accepting T cells graduate from the thymus and escape into the wider world of your body.

White blood cells patrolling your blood rely on physical contact with pathogens to raise the alarm. This usually isn't a problem: loose pathogens floating in your blood will inevitably bump into a white blood cell. But to avoid immune detection, some cunning pathogens – particularly viruses and fungi – squirrel themselves away within your cells, rather than floating loose. Any pathogens hidden inside your cells are hidden from all white blood cells – except for T cells. These thymus-graduated white blood cells can detect intracellular invaders like sniffer dogs detecting packets of cocaine stashed inside a dealer's suitcase. A triggered T cell launches a molecular blitzkrieg, resulting in the implosion, explosion and general chemical kaboom of the infected cell. Nice try, intracellular pathogen.

For those bugs that like to hide inside your cells, eliminating the sniffer dog T cells would be the ultimate invasion strategy. T cells are the only things that stand in the way of undetected entry, replication and massive infection. This is the genius tactic of HIV – human immunodeficiency virus. HIV *specifically infects T cells*. HIV replicates within a T cell then bursts out, destroying the T cell in the process. As more and more T cells are invaded and exploded, the infected person's immune system becomes increasingly weakened. When the T cell count drops below a certain number, the human has AIDS – acquired immunodeficiency syndrome. Death usually follows due to overwhelming infection. Thankfully, modern medication is so effective at halting the T cell attack that HIV is no longer a death sentence, but an entirely manageable chronic disease.

Fiendish foods

When it comes to food allergies, just eight foods account for more than 90 per cent of allergic reactions: peanuts, milk, eggs, tree nuts, fish, shellfish, soybeans and wheat. If you're devising an allergy-friendly menu, pad thai – a mix of noodles, shellfish, peanuts and soy – is a bad choice.

ENDNOTES

1 Blackley, C. H. *Experimental Research on the Causes and Nature of Catarrhus Æstivus*. Oxford Historical Books (1988). First published: Baillière, Tindall and Cox (1873).

2 Bansal, A. S. et al. Dangerous liaison: sexually transmitted allergic reaction to Brazil nuts. *Journal of Investigative Allergology and Clinical Immunology*, 17 (3), 189-191 (2007).

ACNE

**Why pimples crop up on your face, and why acid,
leeches and laxatives won't remove them.**

For as long as humans have had skin, we've had pimples. Acne is a skin disorder that results in outbreaks of pimples. Acne features in writings from Ancient Egyptians, Greeks and Romans. King Tutankhamun's mummified face had acne scars. His tomb contained various honey-based remedies to facilitate his skincare regimen in the afterlife. Hippocrates and Aristotle described the phenomenon of pimples appearing on the face 'when the first beard grows' in adolescence. Roman scholars like Pliny mentioned similar spots with 'peaks of oozing and pain'.

The origin of the word acne isn't clear, much like the complexion of the people who suffer it. One theory goes that 'acne' comes from the Ancient Greeks, who referred to puberty as *acme* ('peak') because it was the peak of a human's growth and development. Writing in the 3rd century AD, Greek historian Cassius claimed that: 'These spots appear on the face at the time of *acme*, as a result of which some laymen call them *acmas*'.[1] Fast-forward 300 years to another Greek writer, Aëtius of Amida who was busy transcribing part of Cassius's work. Perhaps after one ouzo too many, Aëtius made a typo, copying *acnas* instead of *acmas*. This new word infiltrated medical texts and *acmas* became known as *acnas* (acne in the singular) evermore. Maybe. It's a charming story, but many scholars are not convinced by the 'sloppy Aëtius' story.

In 1564, French physician Gorraeus alleged that acne: 'is so called because it does not itch', implying a derivation from the Greek *a + cnao* meaning 'no itch'. In his 1951 essay *The History of Acne*, dermatologist Ronald Grant claims the word acne comes from the Egyptian *aku-t* meaning 'boils, blains, sores, pustules, any inflamed swelling'.[2]

Acne doesn't just bother etymologists: up to 90 per cent of adolescents suffer acne, hence its proper medical name acne *vulgaris* (*vulgaris* being Latin for 'common'). Usually, acne starts in your 'tween years and has all but run its course by your twenties, but some people endure acne into adulthood. In Grant's 1951 essay, he makes a salient observation:

> Acne cannot be regarded as a serious disease or measured
> in terms of life or death, but it has a nuisance value far
> out of proportion to its seriousness, affecting, as it does,
> young people at an age when they are most sensitive to any
> disfigurement.

It could be argued people are sensitive to 'disfigurement' at any age, but his point is fair enough.

*

Humans harbour countless liquid-secreting structures called glands. Lacrimal glands release tears. Mammary glands drip out milk. Mucous, salivary and sweat glands pump out the fluid suggested by their name. When considering acne, it's the sebaceous glands we're interested in. Sebaceous glands lie just under your skin's surface and ooze out an oily mixture called sebum. Rub the side of your nose. The grease you feel is sebum. And grease is the correct term: *sebum* is Latin for grease, related to *sapo* meaning soap (which is also grease, gussied up with perfume and a strong alkali, then portioned into bars and sold at exorbitant prices).

Sebum isn't one substance: it's a concoction of oils including triglycerides, cholesterol, wax esters and the pleasingly named 'squalene' (the main oil in shark livers).

Sebum reaches your skin's surface via holes in the skin called pores. Pores perforate every inch of your skin, providing an escape route not only for sebum, but sweat too. Seeping from your pores, sebum forms an oily coating over your whole body. It lubricates and waterproofs your skin to prevent it becoming cracked and itchy. Its slightly acidic composition also acts as a barrier to disease-causing bacteria, which can't tolerate the low pH.

Most of your pores have a hair poking out of them. Look closely at your forearm. Focus on one hair. See where it seems to emerge from the skin? That's a pore. If you dived down along the hair follicle and looked to the side, you'd see a sebaceous gland seeping sebum around the sub-skin hair. That sebum coats the hair and dribbles out of the overlying pore. Every pore has one of these oil factories – a sebaceous gland – except for the pores on your palms and the soles of your feet.

Wherever you have a sebaceous gland, you can get a pimple.

Making pimples, like making mayonnaise, begins with lots of oil. As the skin lining the follicle naturally sheds, the flakes can become trapped and clog the pore. The determined sebaceous gland keeps exuding its oil. Sebum slowly pools below the skin plug, unable to reach the surface. Bacteria, which already live in vast numbers on your skin, literally strike oil upon finding this plugged greasy well.

Like moths to a flame, white blood cells soon migrate to the battleground to kibosh the bacteria. Dead white blood cells thicken up the soup of sebum, skin flakes and bacteria to form a milky paste – pus. The pus stretches the follicle's walls and this sub-skin volume expansion creates the characteristic pimple bump and pain. Satisfying as it might be, don't attempt to evacuate the pus via squeezing: you'll very likely rupture the follicle and cause scarring.

From a bird's eye view – looking at your face in a mirror – a pus-filled follicle appears as a white dot. Such 'whitehead' pimples have a thin skin layer shielding the pus from the air. If there's no skin cap, the exposed pus turns black due to oxidation (the same reaction that turns a cut apple brown): it's not trapped dirt that gives 'blackheads' their dark colour.

A pimple's pus can spread deeper below the follicle to form a painful pool called a boil (a 'furuncle' in medical lingo). Sometimes several neighbouring follicles develop deep infections, resulting in a cluster of boils. These pools of pus can unite below the skin to form one mega pus lake called a carbuncle. On the surface, the pus oozes from multiple follicles like a family of tiny white worms wriggling out of your skin. Karl Marx, the revolutionary German political theorist, was plagued by carbuncles. Based on scintillating letters he sent to Friedrich Engels, his collaborator on *The Communist Manifesto*, Marx's groin was as inflamed as his political passions:

> I shan't bore you by explaining [the] carbuncles on my posterior and near the penis, the final traces of which are now fading but which made it extremely painful for me to adopt a sitting and hence a writing posture. I am not taking arsenic because it dulls my mind too much and I need to keep my wits about me.[3]

*

Various acne triggers have been touted for millennia. Greek poet Theocritus (c. 300 BC) alleged that pimples on the nose were caused by lying. In the centuries that followed, physicians blamed the spots on tasks requiring mental concentration and heavy blood flow to the head, unrestrained spiritual toil or pain, excessive physical work, a sedentary and idle life, pregnancy, menstruation, and cold and wet climates. The phase 'clutching at straws' springs to mind.

The author of the 1833 text *The Cyclopaedia of Practical Medicine* insisted that acne 'is always very intimately connected with a constipated state of the bowels'.[4] In reality, while both maladies involve blockages – follicles and intestines respectively – that's the extent of their relationship. Other 19th century physicians asserted that 'youthful addiction to the fatal habit of onanism' favoured acne. Onanism, by the way, is masturbation. By 1930 opinion had flipped: now inadequate sexual release caused acne. Doctors referred to acne as 'chastity pustules', believing pimples to be caused by toxin accumulation in the skin of virgins. Further eschewing logic, the treatment wasn't sexual release, but faecal release using laxatives (plus radiation, for good measure).

Then there's the diet blame game. In 1922, dermatologist George MacKee claimed that clear skin required: 'avoiding candy, pastry, soda water, ice cream, chocolate, rich foods, fried foods, cocoa and gravy as a bare minimum plus or minus tea, coffee, alcohol and spices'.[5] In his 1936 book *Cosmetic Dermatology*, Herman Goodman, a dermatologist and syphilologist (which is exactly what it sounds like: a syphilis specialist), added some weirdly specific items to the banned food list: 'starchy foods, bread rolls, noodles, spaghetti, potatoes, oily nuts, chop suey, chow mein, and waffles'.[6] In fact, there is no clear evidence that any specific food item – including chocolate, perhaps the most demonised food when it comes to spots – triggers acne. Feel free to indulge in a plate of gravy-drizzled waffles without worrying about a breakout.

The pseudoscience surrounding acne is probably so strong because people are desperate to blame their spots on something. Alas, there is no single cause of acne. But a few factors can make you more prone to it: plugged follicles, sebaceous glands on steroids, and bacteria-driven inflammation.

Your skin is constantly flaking off into the environment. The skin that lines the sides of your hair follicles is no different. As the central hair grows it should drag any shed skin up to the surface with it, keeping the follicle clean. In people with acne, the skin cells lining the follicle produce too much keratin, a sticky protein naturally found in skin. Excess keratin glues together the skin cells and prevents them from flaking off normally. Gummed-up skin cells, unable to shed, form a plug that traps sebum beneath it.

Acne sufferers have sebaceous glands that squirt out sebum like they're on steroids. Actually, the glands really are on steroids. The exact same steroids that bodybuilders use to bulk up – androgens – are what drive sebaceous glands to produce excess oil. Androgens (such as testosterone) are hormones naturally produced in your body by your adrenal glands, and your ovaries or testicles (see *Balding*, page 66). As well as beefing up your muscles, Adam's apple, and pubic hairs, androgens also enlarge your sebaceous glands. Bigger glands make more sebum. If you're ogling a bodybuilder's washboard abs and notice that they have acne, it's a pretty good clue that the muscles you're admiring aren't 'all natural'. About half of bodybuilders who abuse anabolic steroids break out with acne due to the excess androgens they're injecting. The natural androgen surge with puberty accounts for the development of acne at this time 'when the first beard grows' as the Greeks would say. But acne can strike at a much younger age. Particularly in male babies, rising androgen levels around three months of age can stimulate sebaceous gland growth and result in full-blown acne. Usually the spots clear by the child's first birthday but, just like with adult acne, the scars can be permanent.

Cutibacterium acnes, despite its name, is not a 'cutie': it's the bacterium responsible for much of the inflammation – redness, heat, pain and swelling – that accompanies acne. Healthy skin is covered in harmless bacterial species like *Staphylococcus*. By densely colonising your skin, these friendly bacteria don't leave any room for disease-causing bacteria to set up residence and cause infection. *Cutibacterium acnes* usually belong to the friendly bacteria camp, innocently dwelling in the oil wells provided by hair follicles. But if they become trapped in the follicle (due to a sticky keratin plug, say) the airless environment turns them rogue. Deprived of oxygen, they break down your sebum into fatty acids which trigger inflammation in the surrounding skin. If you're colonised with certain *Cutibacterium acnes* strains, this inflammatory reaction is particularly strong, predisposing you to acne.

*

Historical acne treatments were, to phrase it politely, misguided. Most ancient Romans favoured stinky sulfur baths to clear the skin. But the physician to Roman emperor Theodosius I (347-395 AD) condoned a more convoluted cure:

> Glare at a falling star and, at the very same time the star is still falling from the sky, cover boils with a cloth or anything else to hand. Whilst the star is falling from the sky, boils will fall from your body, yet you must pay special attention not to touch them barehanded or they will pass to your hand.[7]

French surgeon Ambroise Paré claimed that 'many leeches ... attached to the face' would clear the skin, based on the theory that acne resulted from excess facial blood. An 1824 medical text claimed that acne could be cured by sweat-inducing drugs, 'especially when combined with narcotics'.[8] While a sweaty opium binge might distract you from your pimples, it won't do much to treat them. The same text derides other treatments like ceruse (white lead) and Gowland's lotion (containing mercuric chloride) for their 'exorbitant price'. But the problem was more than cost: these heavy metal-containing, skin-blistering treatments were downright dangerous: 'Any misuse caused face skin to be externally and deeply ruined with scars disfiguring the patient's physiognomy more than the disease itself.'[7]

Nowadays we treat acne with creams and tablets that work by unblocking follicles (*not* via squeezing), reducing androgen activity, or killing bacteria. Cleansers can mop up excess sebum, but overzealous scrubbing dehydrates the skin and triggers more sebaceous gland activity. Essentially, if you've got acne you should do the exact opposite of this advice from an 1878 article in *The British Medical Journal*:

> If the sebaceous glands and follicles become overloaded, they should be relieved by pressure between the finger and thumbnail, and by frequent washings with warm water and oatmeal; after which a good rubbing with a flesh-brush will remove the contents of a number of the pimples.[9]

SUMMARY: Acne results from blocked follicles, excess sebum and bacteria-driven inflammation. The trapped paste of sebum, skin cells, bacteria and white blood cells forms pus, which you see through your skin as a pimple.

AND ALSO ...

What's in a name?

The surname Whitehead dates back to Anglo-Saxon tribes in the north of England and Scotland. Having fair hair was noteworthy at the time, hence the descriptive surname. Since dark hair was the norm, 'Blackhead' did not emerge as a surname. It would have been as useless an identifier as the nickname 'two-eyes'. Incidentally, if a medieval Mr Whitehead was troubled by facial whiteheads, he might have blamed it on his parent's failure to rub his face with a urine-soaked cloth as an infant. According to Scottish Highlander folklore, this unsavoury ritual would protect the baby from later developing acne.

G-ow!-land's lotion

John Gowland invented his eponymous lotion in about 1740 as a bespoke remedy for the renowned beauty Elizabeth Chudleigh, the Duchess of Kingston, whose face had developed dark splotches. His basic ingredients were innocent enough: bitter almonds and sugar. But it's the addition of mercuric chloride, a derivative of sulfuric acid, that was problematic. Advertised as a daily scrub, the lotion would chemically peel off the outer layer of the skin, taking any discolouration with it. It worked wonders for the duchess. Her fame and Gowland's sales skyrocketed. For decades, Gowland had a monopoly on skin treatments. In Jane Austen's *Persuasion*, the protagonist Anne's father recommends:

> ... the constant use of Gowland during the spring months. Mrs Clay has been using it at my recommendation, and you see what it has done for her. You see how it has carried away her freckles.

Indeed, it probably had: by chemically obliterating the surface of her face. After Gowland's death in 1776 people began to question whether the skin burning induced by his lotion was such a great idea. In 1810, Northern Irish author John Corrie composed a neat couplet to encapsulate the changing public sentiment:

> There's the lotion of Gowland that flays ladies' faces,
> Distorting the features of our modern graces.[10]

Don't put your finger on it

The Royal Society, founded in London in 1660, is the world's oldest scientific institution. Every year it offers membership to a handful of eminent scientists in recognition of their work. Upon admission, these fellows sign their name in a crimson leather-bound Charter Book. Its hallowed pages feature the autographs of scientific heavyweights including Charles Darwin, Ernest Rutherford, Albert Einstein, Alan Turing and, of course, Isaac Newton. So many sebum-covered fingertips have excitedly underlined Isaac Newton's name that the signature of the poor bloke who signed below him (James Hoare, a forgotten goldsmith) has almost been rubbed off the vellum.

ENDNOTES

1   Goolamali, S. K. & Andison, A. C. The origin and use of the word 'acne'. *British Journal of Dermatology*, 96 (3), 291–294 (1977).

2   Grant, R. N. R. The History of Acne. *Proceedings of the Royal Society of Medicine*, 44 (8), 647–652 (1951).

3   Letter from Karl Marx to Friedrich Engels, 2 April 1867. *Marx and Engels Collected Works Volume 42* p. 350. First published: abridged in *Der Briefwechsel zwischen F. Engels und K. Marx*, Stuttgart (1913) and in full in *MEGA*, Berlin (1930).

4   Forbes, J. et al. *The Cyclopaedia of Practical Medicine: Comprising Treatises on the Nature and Treatment of Disease, Materia Medica and Therapeutics, Medical Jurisprudence, Etc. Etc. Volume 1.* Sherwood, Gilbert, and Piper (1833).

5   Mahmood, N. F. & Shipman, A. R. The age-old problem of acne. *International Journal of Women's Dermatology*, 3 (2), 71–76 (2017).

6   Goodman, H. *Cosmetic Dermatology.* 1st ed. McGraw-Hill (1936).

7   Randazzo, S. D. Acne in the History of Dermatology. *Journal of Applied Cosmetology*, 9 (3) (1991).

8   Good, J. M. *The Study of Medicine: With a Physiological System of Nosology.* Bennett & Walton (1824).

9   Startin, J. The Treatment of Acne. *The British Medical Journal*, 1 (913), 932 (1878).

10 Thompson, C. J. S. *The Mystery and Romance of Alchemy and Pharmacy.* Scientific Press, Limited (1897).

ACKNOWLEDGEMENTS

My patients' curiosity inspired this book; my publishing team's patience saw it come to life.

To my indefatigable editor Geoff Slattery: thank you. You tweaked, nipped and tucked my writing with the deft hand of a gifted plastic surgeon.

Thank you to the team at Hardie Grant for believing in me, and working tirelessly to bring my book to the world.

To neurologists Dr Robb Wesselingh and Dr Emma Foster: as teachers, mentors and role models, you have both fundamentally shaped my medical career. I can't thank you enough for supporting my various research and writing escapades over the years. Your medical proofreading expertise was invaluable.

Above all, thank you to my patients. Your questions and thirst for knowledge motivated me to write this book. Thank you for trusting me, teaching me, inspiring me, and for laughing politely at my jokes.

INDEX